Environmental Toxicology - Understanding, Impact, and Mitigation Strategies for a Sustainable Future

Edited by Suna Sabuncuoğlu and Onur Kenan Ulutaş

Published in London, United Kingdom

Environmental Toxicology - Understanding, Impact, and Mitigation Strategies for a Sustainable Future
http://dx.doi.org/10.5772/intechopen.1008607
Edited by Suna Sabuncuoğlu and Onur Kenan Ulutaş

Contributors
Abiodun Oyeleke, Akinpelu Moronkeji, Beyza Mertaş, Bob-Manuel Chinonso Osuji, Charles Egede Ugwu, Comfort E. Williams, Dipanjali Majumdar, Eduardo Alberto Lopez Maldonado, Emmanuel Tolulope Adegoke, Felipe Dalmazzo Cirinêu, Gassoumi Bouzid, Houcine Barhoumi, İ. İpek Boşgelmez, Izabela da Cunha Bataglioli, Jassem Wannassi, Jiri Adamec, Joshua Olayinka Ajala, José Cavalcante Souza Vieira, Joyce Andrade da Silva, Luane B. Gonçalves Andrade, Luiz Fabrício Zara, Marília Afonso Rabelo Buzalaf, Mohamed Achraf Bouicha, Nicole Jaffrezic-Renault, Olubunmi Esan, Pedro de Magalhães Padilha, Puritan Umeboro, Rachna Jain, Ronaldo de Almeida, Samuel Ayobami Fasogbon, Temidayo Daniel Adeniyi, Tugba Kose, Victor Diego Faria

First published in London, United Kingdom, 2025 by IntechOpen
IntechOpen is the global imprint of INTECHOPEN LIMITED, registered in England and Wales, registration number: 11086078, 167-169 Great Portland Street, London, W1W 5PF, United Kingdom

For EU product safety concerns: IN TECH d.o.o., Prolaz Marije Krucifikse Kozulić 3, 51000 Rijeka, Croatia, info@intechopen.com or visit our website at intechopen.com.

British Library Cataloguing-in-Publication Data
A catalogue record for this book is available from the British Library

Environmental Toxicology - Understanding, Impact, and Mitigation Strategies for a Sustainable Future
Edited by Suna Sabuncuoğlu and Onur Kenan Ulutaş
p. cm.
Print ISBN 978-1-83634-137-6
Online ISBN 978-1-83634-136-9
eBook (PDF) ISBN 978-1-83634-138-3

If disposing of this product, please recycle the paper responsibly.

Meet the editors

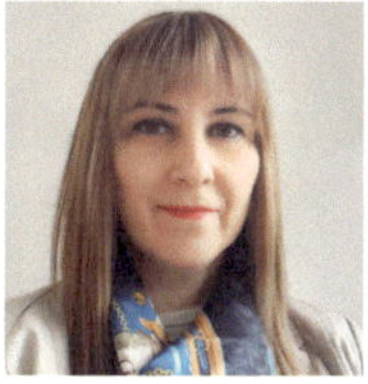

Suna Sabuncuoğlu graduated from Hacettepe University, Faculty of Pharmacy, in 2001. She began working as a research assistant in the Department of Pharmaceutical Toxicology at the same faculty in 2002. She completed her Master's degree in 2005 and her Ph.D. in 2010. During her doctoral studies, she spent one year at the International Agency for Research on Cancer (IARC) in Lyon, France, as an Erasmus student. Following her Ph.D., she conducted postdoctoral research at KU Leuven (Catholic University of Leuven), Belgium. In 2013, she was appointed as a lecturer, and in 2014, she received the title of Associate Professor. In 2022, she was promoted to the rank of Professor. She continues her academic work as a faculty member in the Department of Pharmaceutical Toxicology at Hacettepe University, Faculty of Pharmacy. In addition to her undergraduate and graduate teaching and research activities, she has held various administrative roles. Since 2014, she has been serving as a board member of the Hacettepe University Substance and Alcohol Addiction Research and Application Center. She also serves as the Vice Chair of the Department of Professional Pharmaceutical Sciences and as the Vice Erasmus Coordinator of the Faculty of Pharmacy.

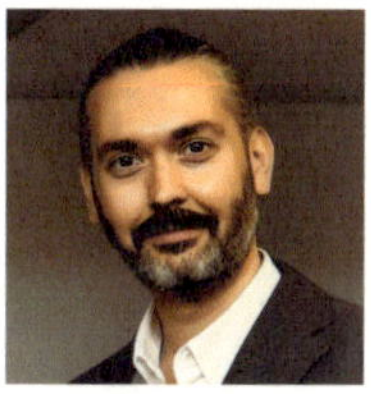

Born in 1982, Onur Kenan Ulutaş serves as Associate Professor and Vice Dean at Gazi University Faculty of Pharmacy. A graduate of TED Ankara College and Gazi University, he completed his Ph.D. in Pharmaceutical Toxicology in 2013, conducting part of his research in Munich with the support of the TÜBİTAK–Helmholtz Doctoral Fellowship. His academic interests span toxicology, pharmacology, and environmental health, with a strong focus on public safety and sustainability. Dr. Ulutaş has authored 89 scientific papers and filed two patents, reflecting both academic depth and innovation. As the founder of the Climate Change and Zero Waste Society (İDESA), he combines scientific insight with social engagement, mentoring students, and fostering collaborative projects at the intersection of science and community.

Contents

Preface

The 21st century has been characterized by profound and often irreversible alterations to the global environment. Some are so subtle as to be additive from the insidious presence of microplastics, endocrine disruptors, persistent organic pollutants, and heavy metals. These pollutants have penetrated every level of biological organization, from cellular machinery to entire ecosystems. The result is a rising wave of health threats, environmental disruptions, and novel chronic diseases whose causes are increasingly referred to as environmental exposures. In the face of these challenges, the field of environmental toxicology has transitioned from the periphery of scientific inquiry to the forefront of planetary health.

Environmental Toxicology – Understanding, Impact, and Mitigation Strategies for a Sustainable Future is born into these imperative times as an interdisciplinary book that embodies the nuance, timeliness, and international importance of environmental toxicology in today's world. It synthesizes novel research and informed commentary from globally and methodologically diverse sources, each striving to expand our understanding of the effects of anthropogenic pollutants on biological systems and how science can react with diagnostic acuity as well as strategic action.

This book brings together contributions that address toxicological problems on molecular, organismal, and ecological scales. Some chapters discuss the molecular mechanisms by which heavy metals, such as mercury, cadmium, arsenic, and lead, disrupt cellular function, antioxidant defense, and hormonal homeostasis. The mechanistic investigations elucidate how environmental exposure is translated into pathophysiological conditions, including diabetes mellitus and Alzheimer's disease, via the induction of oxidative stress, β-cell dysfunction, and neurotoxicity.

Other chapters shift the focus away from environmental and ecotoxicological backgrounds towards technological and methodological innovation. Electrochemical sensor development, functionalized materials, and computational modeling are presented not only as analytical equipment for pollutant detection but also as gateways to real-time environmental monitoring, risk mapping, and data-informed remediation. This book demonstrates how environmental toxicology is increasingly intersecting with materials science, nanotechnology, and artificial intelligence, envisioning a toolkit of early warning, targeted intervention, and eco-friendly solutions.

At a systems level, this book also considers the cascading environmental effects of pollution. Chapters highlight how pollutants degrade biodiversity, destabilize ecosystem services, and erode food and water security, particularly in nations struggling with uncontrolled industry and inadequate waste management infrastructure.

What unifies these disparate contributions is a shared appreciation: that pollutants cannot be treated as separate risks. Their effect is synergistic, their pathways complex, and their effect diffuse, transcending disciplinary borders and geopolitical boundaries.

Environmental toxicology is today as much about prevention and prediction as it is pathology and mechanistic understanding. It demands coordination between disciplines such as analytical chemistry, histopathology, public health, materials engineering, and computational biology. It challenges us to redefine environmental health not merely as a scientific matter, but as a matter of public imperative.

As editors, we believe that *Environmental Toxicology – Understanding, Impact, and Mitigation Strategies for a Sustainable Future* offers analytical rigor and applied value. It is a timely reference for toxicologists, environmental scientists, clinicians, regulators, engineers, and graduate students committed to a solution to the toxicological problems of modern life. Most importantly, it is a sign of a broader shift in the scientific community—toward integrative action from individual observation, toward collective responsibility from fragmented insight.

We take this opportunity to express our sincerest appreciation to all the contributing authors for their intellectual contributions, to the reviewers and co-editors for their thorough assessments, and to the IntechOpen editorial staff for their invaluable support throughout the publication process. We believe that this volume not only educates but also inspires, promoting new scholarship, informing policy discussions, and advancing the international dialogue on environmental justice and ecological resilience.

Dr. Suna Sabuncuoğlu
Professor,
Department of Toxicology,
Hacettepe University,
Ankara, Türkiye

Dr. Onur Kenan Ulutaş
Associate Professor,
Department of Toxicology,
Gazi University,
Ankara, Türkiye

Chapter 1

Histopathological Perspectives on Toxic Environmental Pollutants: Cellular Damage Pathways and Strategic Interventions in Mammalian Systems

Akinpelu Moronkeji, Temidayo Daniel Adeniyi, Samuel Ayobami Fasogbon, Joshua Olayinka Ajala, Emmanuel Tolulope Adegoke, Comfort E. Williams, Abiodun Oyeleke, Charles Egede Ugwu, Olubunmi Esan, Bob-Manuel Chinonso Osuji and Puritan Umeboro

Abstract

Environmental toxicants (ETs) are pervasive and often exert synergistic effects that pose significant health risks to mammalian systems. Major pollutants such as airborne particulate matter ($PM_{2.5}/PM_{1.0}$), heavy metals, and various classes of agricultural pesticides continue to contribute to environmental degradation and disease burden. These toxicants originate from diverse sources, including battery manufacturing, metal plating, phosphate fertilisers, plastic stabilisers, plumbing systems, fossil fuel combustion, and intensive agricultural practices. A systematic evaluation of their public health implications is critical for informing policy and intervention. This chapter explores the mechanisms of toxicity of these environmental pollutants, highlighting their cellular and histopathological effects on mammalian tissues while proposing intervention strategies to safeguard human health and the ecosystem.

Keywords: environmental pollution, histopathology, mammalian system, oxidative stress, public health

1. Introduction

1.1 Overview of major environmental pollutants

Environmental toxicants (ETs) are widespread contaminants that can adversely affect mammalian health as toxicants bioaccumulate in organs, inducing oxidative stress and disrupting enzymatic functions, which can lead to DNA damage, thus predisposing to cancer and various types of metabolic diseases [1]. The exposure to ETs, like pesticides, organic pollutants, and heavy metals, can lead to multi- and transgenerational effects on fertility [2]. Reports have highlighted the integral role of the NLRP3 inflammasome in mediating the inflammatory responses triggered by ETs, contributing to organ damage and autoimmune diseases [3].

1.1.1 Airborne particulate matter ($PM_{2.5}$, $PM_{1.0}$)

Particulate matter (PM) is a complex mixture of solid particles and liquid droplets of varying sizes and content suspended in air. Sources include natural phenomena like volcanic eruptions and anthropogenic activities like industrial processes and vehicular emissions [4]. Indoor PM concentrations can exceed outside levels originating from activities such as cooking and smoking [5]. Fine ($PM_{2.5}$) and ultrafine particulate (UFP) matter ($PM_{1.0}$) represent considerable health concerns, particularly to the respiratory system and infant development.

They can penetrate deeply into the lungs, causing respiratory disorders as well as systemic effects [6]. Exposure to $PM_{2.5}$ causes pro-inflammatory cytokine release, DNA damage, and the buildup of cancer metabolites [7]. $PM_{2.5}$ exposure triggers pro-inflammatory cytokine release, DNA damage, and cancer metabolite accumulation [7]. PM exposure in the developing brain promotes oxidative stress, inflammation, and blood-brain barrier disruption, potentially leading to neurodevelopmental problems such as attention deficit disorders and autism spectrum disorders [8].

1.1.2 Heavy metals

Heavy metals are elements that naturally occur and have atomic weights and densities that are at least five times greater than those of water [9]. Although elements like copper are considered essential trace nutrients for biological functions, other heavy metals such as lead (Pb), cadmium (Cd), and mercury (Hg) are known for their high toxicity and tendency to bioaccumulate. These metals can infiltrate the environment through air, water, soil, and food chains, posing serious threats to human and ecological health by contributing to both acute and long-term health complications [10–12]. Anthropogenic activities associated with industrial, agricultural, and technological applications have significantly elevated the widespread presence of pollutants in the environment [13, 14]. Reports have documented the deleterious impact of heavy metal exposure, including toxicity associated with multiple organ damage, and they are classified as human carcinogens as they accumulate in environmental matrices and can enter the food chain, leading to bioaccumulation in humans and causing various diseases, including cancer [9, 15]. Lead interferes with enzymatic systems and calcium signalling, particularly affecting children's developing nervous systems, while cadmium accumulates in the kidneys and liver, causing nephrotoxicity and increasing the risk of cancer [16, 17]. This mechanism of exerting toxicity is by strongly coordinating with biological molecules, replacing essential metals in proteins and enzymes, and inducing oxidative stress. Treatment strategies for metal poisoning often involve chelation therapy, especially in acute cases [18, 19].

1.1.3 Pesticides (pyrethroids, organophosphates, carbamates, organochlorines)

Both synthetic and natural pesticides are widely employed in agriculture and public health for pest control, but their extensive application has led to environmental contamination and potential toxic effects on various organisms [20–22]. Conventional pesticides can persist in the environment for decades, harming non-target species and ecosystems. These chemicals accumulate in the food chain, affecting human health by damaging organs, causing diseases, and potentially leading to death [23]. Biopesticides, derived from natural sources, offer a safer alternative with reduced environmental impact and lower toxicity to humans and beneficial organisms [24]. Pyrethroids, synthetic analogues of natural pyrethrins, exert neurotoxic effects by targeting sodium channels in nerve cells. Their exposure has been linked to oxidative stress, inflammation, and mitochondrial dysfunction, which could contribute to neurodegenerative diseases like Parkinson's [25]. Pyrethroids also reduce antioxidant levels, induce kidney toxicity, alter immune responses, and disrupt carbohydrate and lipid metabolism, increasing the risk of obesity [26, 27]. Pyrethroids are classified based on their chemical structure and symptomology, with Type I and Type II compounds exhibiting different effects on sodium channel currents and neuronal excitability [28]. Organophosphates (OPs) are highly toxic compounds widely used as pesticides and in other applications. Their principal mechanism of toxicity is the inhibition of acetylcholinesterase, leading to acetylcholine accumulation in cholinergic synapses [29]. This can cause cholinergic crisis, characterised by muscle twitching, respiratory distress, and potentially death. Acute exposure can trigger status epilepticus, resulting in long-term brain damage if uncontrolled [30]. Clinical manifestations include cholinergic excess, nicotinic effects, cardiac complications, and respiratory failure, with management involving resuscitation, atropine administration, and oxime therapy [31]. Organochlorines, particularly dichlorodiphenyltrichloroethane (DDT) and its metabolites, are considered persistent organic pollutants (POPs) due to their environmental persistence, bioaccumulative potential, and toxicity [32, 33]. Furthermore, beyond reproductive toxicity, these compounds have also been implicated in the disruption of the central nervous system (CNS), immune function, and metabolic processes [34].

1.2 Sources and pathways of exposure

1.2.1 Industrial emissions

Industrial activities are significant sources of environmental contaminants, particularly heavy metals and chemical pollutants. Heavy metals like mercury, lead, and cadmium, released from industries such as battery manufacturing, can contaminate air, soil, and water. These pollutants can enter the human body *via* inhalation, ingestion, or dermal absorption, leading to a range of health problems such as cancer, cardiovascular disorders, and neurological impairments [35]. Likewise, the combustion of fossil fuels in industrial settings releases polycyclic aromatic hydrocarbons (PAHs), volatile organic compounds (VOCs), and other airborne contaminants, which are associated with respiratory illnesses, central nervous system dysfunction, and additional adverse health effects [36].

1.2.2 Agricultural runoff and pesticide usage

Modern agricultural practices heavily rely on chemical fertilisers and pesticides, which can contaminate water resources through runoff and seepage [37]. Organophosphate pesticides, in particular, are widely used and can inhibit acetylcholinesterase, leading to neurological disorders [38]. These agrochemicals remain persistent in the environment, accumulate in aquatic organisms, and subsequently enter the food chain, ultimately posing health risks to humans. Pesticide exposure can occur *via* several channels, including contaminated food, water, and direct contact, resulting in developmental defects, skin disorders, and potential carcinogenic effects [23, 39]. The presence of these chemicals in the aquatic ecosystem has caused population declines in fish and other species, disrupting food webs [40].

1.2.3 Environmental persistence and bioaccumulation

Persistent organic pollutants (POPs) are synthetic compounds that are resistant to degradation and persist for extended periods within the environment [41]. These

S/N	Toxicant	Modulatory mechanism
1.	Arsenic (As)	Inhibits mitochondrial enzymes such as pyruvate dehydrogenase and succinate dehydrogenase, hence disrupting cellular respiration. It causes oxidative stress, disrupts DNA repair pathways, and promotes apoptosis, making it both carcinogenic and hazardous to many organs, including the skin, liver, and kidneys [43, 44].
2.	Lead (Pb)	Lead interferes with several enzymatic pathways and mimics calcium. It causes long-term neurotoxicity, anaemia, and developmental abnormalities in children by interfering with the release of neurotransmitters, preventing haem synthesis by blocking enzymes such as δ-aminolevulinic acid dehydratase, and building up in bone [45, 46].
3.	Mercury (Hg)	Mercury exposure can lead to glutathione depletion, increased reactive oxygen species (ROS) formation, and damage to DNA and protein structures. In the nervous system, Hg alters neurotransmitter receptors, cytoskeleton, and synaptic proteins, disrupting synaptic structure and function. Methylmercury, an organic form, is particularly neurotoxic, as it can cross the blood-brain barrier and affect multiple molecular pathways, including glutamate signalling and the antioxidant [47–49].
4.	Cadmium (Cd)	Primarily targets the liver and kidneys, inducing oxidative stress and inflammation [50, 51]. Cadmium exposure leads to elevated ROS levels, DNA damage, and inhibition of DNA repair mechanisms. Chronic exposure can result in various cancers, osteoporosis, and respiratory issues. Exposure is also linked to mitochondrial dysfunction, epigenetic changes, and the disruption of essential metals [52, 53].
5.	Benzene (C_6H_6)	Benzene is a known haematotoxic and leukaemogenic chemical that targets haematopoietic stem cells (HSCs), causing haematological disorders and cancer. When metabolised, benzene produces toxic intermediates that accumulate in the bone marrow, generating ROS and damaging haematopoietic progenitor cells [54].
6.	Particulate matter ($PM_{2.5}$ and $PM_{1.0}$)	PM can penetrate deep into lung alveoli, entering the bloodstream, causing systemic inflammation, oxidative stress, and endothelial dysfunction by generating ROS, activating pro-inflammatory pathways, and impairing mitochondrial function, resulting in increased morbidity and mortality and contributing to cardiovascular diseases, respiratory disorders, and neurodegenerative conditions [36, 55–59].
7.	Organophosphate pesticides	Organophosphates (OPs) are potent neurotoxins that primarily exert their toxicity by predominantly inhibiting acetylcholinesterase (AChE), resulting in excessive accumulation of acetylcholine at synapses. This results in a cholinergic crisis, which involves continuous activation of muscles, glands, and the CNS, resulting in seizures and respiratory paralysis [30, 60–62].

Table 1.
Toxicodynamic mechanisms of some environmental contaminants on the mammalian systems.

lipophilic substances bioaccumulate in living organisms and biomagnify through food chains, posing serious threats to human health and ecosystems [42]. POPs include pesticides, industrial chemicals, and byproducts [41]. Their ubiquitous prevalence in various environmental compartments, including water, soil, and air, facilitates long-range transport and global distribution. **Table 1** shows the toxicodynamic mechanism of selected environmental toxicants affecting the mammalian system.

2. Diagnostic relevance of histopathological evaluation in environmental toxicology

Histopathological evaluation remains integral in the diagnosis and assessment of tissue alterations induced by toxic environmental pollutants, as microscopic examination of tissue architecture provides critical insight into cellular and subcellular changes resulting from chronic or acute exposure to pollutants such as heavy metals, persistent organic pollutants (POPs), particulate matter, and volatile organic compounds [57, 63, 64]. In non-clinical toxicological evaluations, histopathology provides critical insight into organ-specific toxicity and carcinogenicity by identifying characteristic morphological alterations such as inflammation, necrosis, fibrosis, hyperplasia, and neoplasia, which serve as definitive evidence of pollutant-induced tissue damage [65]. Furthermore, while this diagnostic approach not only buttresses the link between exposure and disease manifestation, it also aids in determining the severity, reversibility, and pathogenesis of toxic insults on the mammalian system. Within environmental toxicology, histopathological analysis serves as an indispensable tool for validating experimental findings, guiding regulatory decisions, and advancing public health risk assessments [66]. For cancer detection, histopathology provides accurate identification of malignancies, guides tumour grading and staging, and detects biomarkers that influence treatment decisions [67].

2.1 Role of histopathology in detecting early and chronic tissue damage

Environmental toxicological studies often require the use of selected histopathological techniques for detecting early-stage cellular changes, inflammatory responses, degenerative alterations, and precancerous lesions [68, 69]. These methods enable detailed examination of tissue architecture and cellular morphology, allowing for accurate diagnosis and treatment planning in various conditions, including cervical cancer [70, 71]. While conventional bright-field microscopy has limitations, advanced imaging techniques can offer high-resolution 3D volumetric imaging of tissue structures at the nanometre scale, enhancing cancer pathobiology research [72]. Furthermore, machine learning approaches, including both classical and deep learning techniques, are increasingly being applied to histopathological image analysis, improving diagnostic accuracy and efficiency [73]. Despite significant progress, challenges remain in standardising techniques and scoring patterns to ensure reliability across different contexts. For instance, histopathological examination remains the gold standard for diagnosing and staging liver diseases, particularly non-alcoholic steatohepatitis (NASH). It allows for accurate assessment of disease severity, including steatosis, inflammation, and fibrosis, which are crucial for determining prognosis and guiding treatment. While non-invasive methods are advancing, they cannot yet match the detailed information provided by liver histology [74]. However, the integration of digital pathology and artificial intelligence (AI) is revolutionising histopathological analysis, as AI-based technologies can automate slide evaluation, eliminate observer subjectivity, and extract hidden patterns relevant to disease progression, further offering potential improvements in disease grading and prognostication across various organ systems [75].

2.2 Relevance in toxicological screening and health surveillance

Histopathology is particularly significant in toxicological investigations, providing vital insights into the effects of chemicals and drugs on biological tissues. It is essential for identifying target organ toxicity, evaluating dose-response relationships, and characterising mechanisms of action at the cellular level. Histopathological examination is particularly important in non-clinical toxicological evaluations, offering data on organ-specific toxicity and carcinogenicity. Recent advancements in digital pathology and deep learning have created opportunities to improve workflow efficiency and provide more objective assessments in toxicologic histopathology [76]. Mechanistic toxicology, which studies molecular, biochemical, and cellular interactions leading to toxicological effects, relies heavily on histopathology to evaluate health risks and safety in pharmacological and environmental toxicology. This approach has led to the discovery of biomarkers for monitoring potential toxicity progression following exposure to various substances [5]. In occupational health, histologic evaluation of dust burden in lung tissues can reveal environmental/occupational aetiologies that may otherwise be misclassified as idiopathic pulmonary fibrosis. Minimal criteria for dust characterisation in lung biopsies have been proposed to improve diagnosis accuracy [77].

2.3 Histopathological alterations in mammalian organs

2.3.1 Respiratory system

Globally, air pollution significantly affects human health, particularly the respiratory system. Exposure to fine PM is linked to reduced lung function, lower quality of life, and increased risks of acute respiratory infections, asthma, COPD, and lung cancer [78, 79]. Approximately 30% of respiratory diseases have been linked to personal exposure to high concentrations of ambient particulate matter (PM), which consists of tiny solid particles or liquid droplets suspended in the air [6]. These particles, originating from both human activities and natural sources, represent a heterogeneous mixture of various sizes and chemical compositions. Common constituents include sulphur dioxide, nitrogen dioxide, salts, carbonaceous materials, VOCs, polycyclic aromatic hydrocarbons (PAHs), and endotoxin [80, 81]. Exposure to PM can induce significant lung injury through multiple mechanisms. Generally, PM fractions of larger sizes (> PM2.5) deposit in the upper airways through impaction, while lesser fractions (< PM2.5) seep deeper into the lower airways and alveoli, depending on flow rates and diffusion, and could be transported to other regions through the bloodstream after inhalation [82]. Furthermore, pulmonary fibrosis is promoted by PM2.5 *via* the induction of mitochondrial dysfunction and epithelial-mesenchymal transition in alveolar type II cells [83]. Short-term exposure triggers inflammatory responses, particularly involving macrophages and neutrophils, but the lung can initiate repair mechanisms [84]. Exposure to $PM_{2.5}$ also leads to oxidative stress, downregulation of antioxidant pathways, and damage to alveolar type II cells [85]. The NLRP3 inflammasome in macrophages plays a crucial role in $PM_{2.5}$-induced lung injury by mediating pyroptosis and exacerbating inflammation, oxidative stress, and apoptosis [86]. PM2.5 causes oxidative stress in human lung tissue and BEAS-2B cells by activating enzymes such as nicotinamide adenine dinucleotide phosphate (NADPH), quinine oxidoreductase (NQO), haem oxygenase-1 (HO-1), and glutamate-cysteine ligase catalytic subunit (GCLC). These enzymes stimulate Nrf2 *via* transmitting signals from phosphatidylinositol-4,5-biphosphate 3-kinase, which are linked to Nrf2 signalling, while also downregulating Nrf2-related transcription factors and increasing IL-8 gene expression [87, 88]. Additionally, PM2.5 activates the oxidative stress-related IL-6/AKT/STAT3/NF-κB signalling pathway, which upregulates intercellular adhesion molecule-1 (ICAM-1) expression in vascular endothelial cells. This cascade contributes to oxidative stress, DNA damage, and eventual death of pulmonary epithelial cells [89].

2.3.2 Alveolar damage, bronchial inflammation, fibrosis

Particulate matter exposure adversely affects the respiratory system *via* oxidative stress induction and inflammation by ROS generation, further leading to the activation of immune responses involving cytokines and chemokines, creating a cycle of inflammation that can lead to apoptosis, necrosis, and widespread tissue damage, which are processes central to the pathogenesis of asthma, COPD, and other pulmonary disorders, highlighting the need for stringent protection and regulatory measures [90–92]. Histologically, PM causes alveolar wall thickening, inflammatory cell infiltration, and pulmonary fibrosis [93]. PM induces oxidative stress, triggering inflammatory responses and fibrotic changes through pathways involving TXNIP/NF-κB and TGF-β/Smad3. These mechanisms contribute to epithelial-to-mesenchymal transition, increasing fibronectin production and promoting fibrosis. Chronic PM exposure results in bronchiolitis, characterised by fibrosis and distortion of small airways, particularly the distal membranous and respiratory bronchioles. Furthermore, exposure disrupts intracellular calcium homeostasis, a key regulator of cellular processes. Elevated intracellular Ca^{2+} levels, triggered by ROS and lipid peroxidation, activate inflammatory pathways and further ROS production, creating a vicious cycle of cellular damage [94].

2.3.3 Hepatic system

2.3.3.1 Hepatocellular degeneration and steatosis

Non-alcoholic fatty liver disease (NAFLD), a multifactorial disorder characterised by fat accumulation in the liver, is one of the most common chronic liver conditions globally. Environmental toxicants like heavy metals and organic pollutants play a significant role in the development of metabolic dysfunction-associated steatotic liver disease [95, 96]. Acute exposure to pollutants like PM triggers low-grade inflammation in the lungs and liver, marked by elevated pro-inflammatory cytokines, as shown in **Figure 1**. Key molecular pathways involved include JNKs-AP1, NF-κB, and TLR4. Additionally, pollutant exposure disrupts peroxisome proliferator-activated receptor (PPAR) activity, impairing lipid and glucose metabolism [98]. Exposure to Cd, Pb, As, and Hg is associated with increased risk of non-alcoholic fatty liver disease (NAFLD) and altered liver injury markers [99]. These metals induce hepatic lipid accumulation by activating lipogenesis and inhibiting fatty acid β-oxidation through various signalling pathways [17]. Perfluorooctane sulfonate (PFOS), an organic

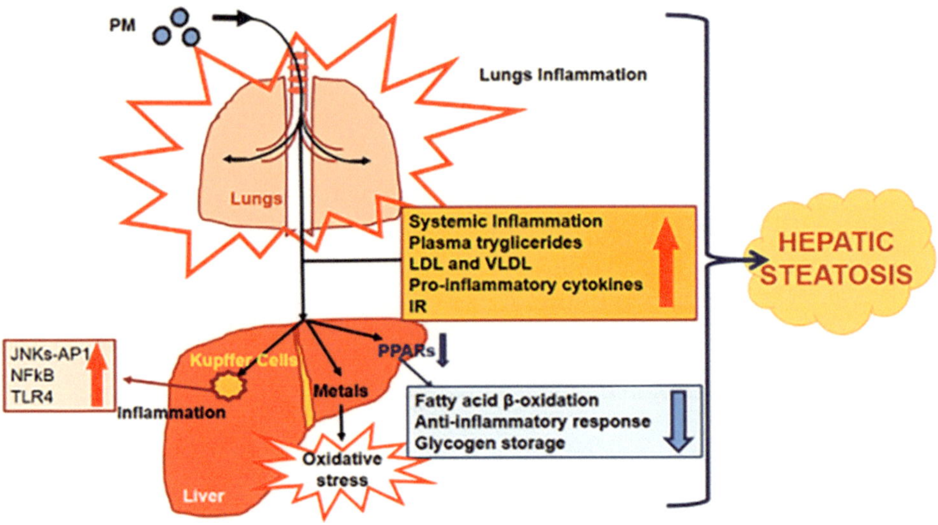

Figure 1.
Diagram of inhaled particulate matter promoting hepatic steatosis [97].

pollutant, promotes hepatic steatosis by inhibiting AMP-activated protein kinase (AMPK) phosphorylation, leading to increased acetyl-CoA carboxylase activity and reduced fatty acid oxidation. Endocrine-disrupting chemicals (EDCs) interfere with nuclear receptors, disrupt hormonal signalling, and impair mitochondrial function, contributing to MASLD development [100]. Occupational exposure to toxicants is also implicit in MASLD progression to advanced chronic liver disease and hepatocellular carcinoma [101].

2.3.4 Renal system

Heavy metals like Pb, Cr, Cd, Hg, and As pose significant health risks because of their persistence in the environment and potential to contaminate soil and drinking water [102]. Human exposure commonly arises from industrial activities such as mining, tanning, textile dyeing (chromium), battery production (cadmium), pesticide and fertiliser use (mercury), and smelting processes (arsenic) [103]. These metals can accumulate in the body and damage vital organs. Toxicity is determined by factors such as the absorbed dose, the route of exposure, and whether the exposure was acute or chronic. Toxic effects are largely mediated by oxidative stress caused by free radical generation, resulting in cellular injury and various health disorders [104]. Kupffer cells (KCs) play an integral role in the progression of liver diseases such as alcohol-associated liver disease (ALD) and non-alcoholic fatty liver disease (NAFLD) [95, 96]. When activated, KCs release pro-inflammatory cytokines and chemokines, contributing to liver inflammation and fibrosis [96, 105]. They interact with hepatic stellate cells, promoting their activation and subsequent fibrosis. Interestingly, KCs can also transdifferentiate into fibrocytes, directly participating in liver fibrosis. Activation of pattern recognition receptors on KCs and other liver cells causes the generation of pro-inflammatory and pro-fibrotic factors, further exacerbating liver damage [105].

2.3.4.1 Glomerular and tubular injury due to Cd and Pb exposure

Cadmium and lead are non-essential heavy metals with no physiological function in humans and are recognised for their high toxicological significance, with chronic exposure, even at low environmental levels, strongly linked to nephrotoxicity, elevated risk of chronic kidney disease (CKD), and metabolic disorders such as diabetes mellitus [106]. These metals predominantly accumulate in the proximal renal tubules, causing structural damage such as tubular atrophy, interstitial fibrosis, and glomerular injury. Chronic elevated Pb exposure can lead to irreversible kidney changes such as interstitial fibrosis, tubular atrophy, glomerular sclerosis, and, eventually, renal failure. Co-exposure to Cd and Pb has been shown to enhance nephrotoxicity, with Cd being the principal cause of renal tubular destruction and Pb amplifying Cd's effects [106]. Pb induces oxidative stress indirectly by increasing the concentration of free Fe, which acts as a Fenton's metal. The elevated Fe in the blood occurs due to the Pb displacement from the haemoglobin molecule (plumbemia). Pb mimics and displaces essential cations (Ca^{2+}, Zn^{2+}, Cu^{2+}, and Mn^{2+}), which are crucial cofactors of antioxidant enzymes, thus reducing their activity by elevating oxidative stress in the tissues. In addition, Cd primarily enters the body *via* ingestion of contaminated food, inhalation of tobacco smoke, and inhalation of polluted air. Smokers, for instance, have been found to exhibit Cd blood levels 4–5 times higher than non-smokers [107]. Once absorbed into the bloodstream, Cd binds to albumin and is transported to the liver, where it induces the synthesis of metallothionein (MT). This leads to the formation of cadmium-metallothionein (CdMT) complexes [108]. Cadmium's long biological half-life of about 25 years leads to its progressive accumulation in renal tissue. Although only a portion of inhaled (10–50%) and ingested (5–10%) Cd is absorbed, long-term exposure poses significant health risks [109].

2.3.5 Nervous system

2.3.5.1 Neurotoxic effects of chronic pesticide exposure: Mechanisms and implications

Chronic pesticide exposure, particularly to organophosphates, pyrethroids, and fungicides, has been increasingly associated with neurological and neurodegenerative disorders, such as Alzheimer's disease, Parkinson's disease, and amyotrophic lateral sclerosis (ALS). These chemicals induce oxidative stress, disrupt neurotransmission, and cause neuronal damage in brain regions such as the hippocampus, corpus striatum, cerebral cortex, and cerebellum [110, 111]. Pesticides act through multiple neurotoxic pathways. They inhibit acetylcholinesterase activity, impair mitochondrial function by disrupting the electron transport chain (ETC) and oxidative phosphorylation (OXPHOS), and elevate ROS, resulting in oxidative damage [112]. Some pesticides, such as rotenone, DDT, and DDE, also activate NADPH oxidases, further promoting ROS accumulation and neuroinflammation [113]. Many pesticides can cross the blood-brain barrier, leading to direct neural damage and gliosis, which is directly associated with injury or neurodegeneration [114]. Pyrethroids, in particular, have been implicated in behavioural impairments, Tau hyperphosphorylation, and neurofibrillary tangle formation consistent with Alzheimer's pathology. Fungicides at environmentally relevant doses (e.g., 0.1 μg/L in drinking water) have been shown to promote β-amyloid ($A\beta_{1-42}$) fibrillogenesis, elevate BACE1 levels, reduce neprilysin activity, and increase cerebral amyloid deposition, contributing to cognitive decline and cerebral amyloid angiopathy [115, 116]. The cumulative neurotoxic effects of chronic pesticide exposure are mediated through oxidative stress, mitochondrial dysfunction, neuroinflammation, and dysregulation of Aβ and tau-related pathways, all of which compromise neuronal integrity and brain function [8, 117]. This evidence underscores the need for urgent, stricter regulatory measures and neuroprotective strategies, particularly for at-risk populations such as agricultural workers and residents in farming regions. Additionally, while certain heavy metals are well-established contributors to the development and exacerbation of various diseases, emerging pollutants have also been increasingly associated with histopathological alterations, as documented in **Table 2**. **Figure 2** also highlights the potential neuropathological mechanisms associated with pesticide exposure.

Pollutant type	Organ affected	Histopathological findings	Reference
Polystyrene microplastics	Lung	Cytotoxic and inflammatory	[118]
Polystyrene microplastics	Placenta	Oxidative stress, mitochondrial swelling, and trophoblast degeneration	[119]
Polyethylene microplastics	Ileum	Villous atrophy, hyperplasia of goblet cells, nuclear pyknosis, and heightened immunoreactivity of p53	[120]
Polystyrene microspheres	Liver, kidney, brain	Disruptions in amino acid metabolism, oxidative stress pathways, and pro-inflammatory cytokine expression	[121]
Titanium dioxide nanoparticles	Liver	Fibrosis, inflammation, and hepatocellular necrosis	[122]
Glyphosate agrochemical	Brain	Increased immunoreactivity	[60]

Table 2.
Summary of histopathological effects of selected emerging pollutants.

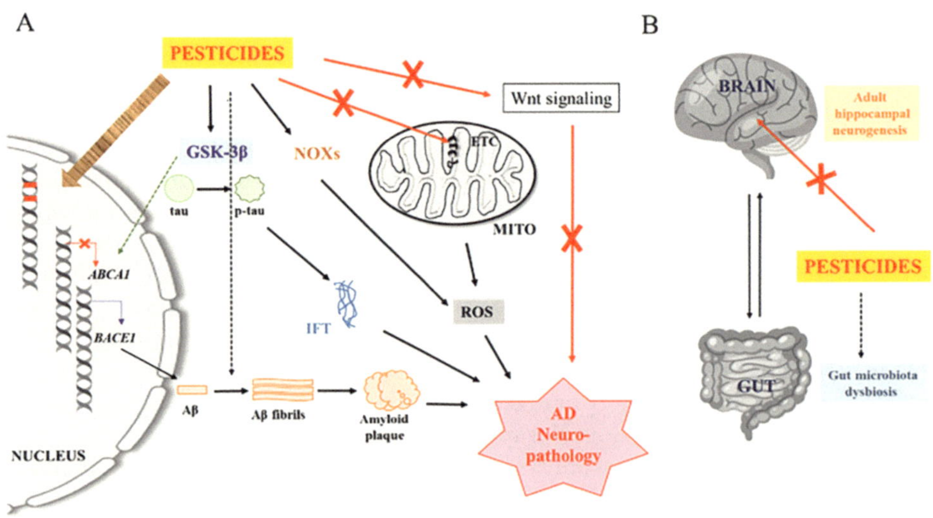

Figure 2.
Diagram of potential neuropathological mechanisms of pesticides [117].

3. Environmental and regulatory controls

3.1 Phasing out persistent organic pollutants (POPs)

Persistent organic pollutants (POPs) are synthetic toxicants known for their environmental persistence, bioaccumulative potential, and long-range transport. Derived primarily from industrial chemicals and agricultural pesticides, these compounds pose considerable health and ecological risks due to their high toxicity and resistance to degradation [123]. Common examples include dichlorodiphenyltrichloroethane (DDT), polychlorinated biphenyls (PCBs), and dioxins. In humans, exposure mainly occurs through the intake of contaminated food, especially fatty animal-based products, where POPs accumulate in adipose tissues. Secondary exposures may occur *via* drinking contaminated water or dermal contact. Importantly, POPs can cross the placenta and be transferred to infants through breast milk. Despite this, global health agencies emphasise that the benefits of breastfeeding continue to outweigh the potential risks posed by POPs [124, 125].

Histopathological studies in laboratory models have demonstrated typical tissue damage from POP exposures, such as hepatocellular ballooning, renal tubular vacuolisation, and aberrant immune infiltration [125]. Additionally, zebrafish larvae exposed to realistic human-relevant POP mixtures exhibited cartilage malformations and impaired bone mineralisation, largely mediated by interference with nuclear receptor signalling pathways, including androgen, vitamin D, and retinoic acid receptors [126].

3.2 Air and water quality regulation

Air and water pollution are major global public health challenges. Airborne pollutants like $PM_{2.5}$, VOCs, SO_2, and NO_x largely stem from fossil fuel combustion, industrial processes, and vehicle emissions, while water contaminants such as Pb, Cd, As, Hg, and pesticides are linked to activities like mining, agriculture, and improper waste disposal [127]. The variable chemical makeup of these pollutants, including trace metals, inorganic salts, and organic matter, contributes to oxidative stress, inflammation, and organ damage. $PM_{2.5}$, for instance, can cause alveolar injury and fibrosis, while chronic exposure to waterborne heavy metals leads to renal and hepatic toxicity and DNA damage [128, 129]. Many developing and underdeveloped countries lack comprehensive regulatory policies on air and water quality. In contrast, developed nations like the United States have established frameworks such as the Clean Air Act and the Safe Drinking Water Act, which enable the Environmental Protection Agency (EPA) to regulate pollutants. Additionally, the World Health Organisation (WHO) offers global guidelines to protect vulnerable populations [130]. However, enforcement and implementation vary widely across regions, with significant disparities between high-income and low-resource settings [127]. Technological advancements such as satellite-based environmental monitoring, real-time air quality sensors, and community-level water testing have greatly enhanced pollution surveillance [131].

3.3 Biomedical intervention

3.3.1 Use of antioxidants and chelators

Environmental toxicants frequently induce excessive production of ROS, leading to oxidative stress that compromises mitochondrial function and causes structural damage to lipids, proteins, and DNA. This oxidative injury manifests histologically as cytoplasmic vacuolisation, necrosis, and apoptotic cell death [56, 132, 133]. Antioxidant therapies, particularly N-acetylcysteine (NAC), help restore redox balance and protect cellular structures, with evidence showing NAC's efficacy in reversing cadmium-induced renal and mitochondrial damage [134]. Particulate matter and ultrafine particulates (UFPs), rich in trace metals and organics, further aggravate systemic oxidative stress and inflammation [135].

Chelation therapy using agents like ethylenediaminetetraacetic acid (EDTA) and dimercaptosuccinic acid (DMSA) enhances metal excretion and improves histopathological outcomes in metal-exposed individuals but must be applied carefully to prevent loss of essential minerals. Oxidative injury is often amplified by pollutants such as nitrogen dioxide, ozone, and polycyclic aromatic hydrocarbons (PAHs), which promote ROS generation through redox reactions like the Fenton reaction. These free radicals disrupt mitochondrial function, fragment DNA, and activate pro-inflammatory pathways such as NF-κB and MAPK [135]. A crucial regulator of antioxidant defence is nuclear factor erythroid 2-related factor 2 (Nrf2), which controls the expression of detoxification and cytoprotective genes [136]. Nrf2 activation mitigates oxidative damage induced by environmental pollutants, while its deficiency heightens susceptibility to cytotoxicity and inflammation [137]. This pathway is increasingly recognised as a promising therapeutic target for pollution-induced tissue injury. Recent findings by Issa et al. [138] demonstrate that chronic exposure to thiamethoxam (TMX), a widely used neonicotinoid pesticide, causes dose-dependent liver and kidney injury, marked by suppressed antioxidant activity, increased lipid peroxidation, and DNA fragmentation. Immunomodulatory drugs have shown efficacy in pollutant-induced injury. For example, corticosteroids have been used in murine models to normalise alveolar architecture and reduce lung inflammation triggered by PM *via* suppression of IL-1β and TNF-α [139, 140]. These interventions may reduce mucosal damage and chronic inflammation, although further clinical validation is required.

3.4 Public health strategies

3.4.1 Biomonitoring and health surveillance

Biomonitoring (BM) is a useful technique in exposure assessment since it tracks exposure to harmful contaminants and their effects in exposed subjects' bodily fluids. This method evaluates the overall absorbed dose of xenobiotic chemicals while accounting for individual factors such as age, gender, and physiological conditions, as well as the numerous exposure sources arising from the environment and personal habits (such as diet and cigarette smoking). Using a non-invasive matrix, the measurement of chemicals in urine is a reliable method for obtaining exposure profiles at low environmental levels [141]. According to Viegas et al. [142], BM includes exposure from every source. It can be used to evaluate the efficacy of current risk-management strategies and find unintended and unforeseen exposures. Biomonitoring involves the assessment of chemicals and their metabolites within the human body, typically by analysing exhaled breath condensate, blood, urine, hair, or breast milk. It offers a combined indicator of the degree of chemical exposure from several exposure pathways.

DOI: http://dx.doi.org/10.5772/intechopen.1012228

3.4.2 Risk communication and community-based intervention

Effective risk communication remains essential for community-based interventions addressing environmental pollution, as it helps the public understand the harmful effects of chemical contamination. Success relies on delivering culturally sensitive, locally tailored messages that consider community demographics, history, and sociocultural factors [143]. Understanding community perceptions and knowledge sources enhances the relevance and impact of these strategies, further fostering trust, engagement, and more effective responses to environmental health risks [144]. In several low- and middle-income countries (LMICs), inadequate data from poor waste management and infrastructural limitations hinder accurate risk assessment, which negatively impacts effective communication that is not only crucial for guiding public health actions but also for reducing anxiety, encouraging behaviour change, fostering trust, and promoting environmental justice [145–147]. Furthermore, adequate engagement of the community further strengthens the interpretation of scientific findings, facilitates message dissemination, and ensures policies reflect public needs, which is an approach endorsed by the WHO's Helsinki Statement [148]. Involving local stakeholders in health policy development increases its relevance and sustainability [149]. Also, multisectoral interventions spanning transport, urban planning, industry, agriculture, and personal behaviour are increasingly employed to reduce pollution exposure, often supported by legislation and public-private partnerships, while behavioural interventions remain essential for minimising personal exposure risks [150].

4. Conclusion

The ongoing rise in industrialisation, urban development, and global expansion continues to escalate environmental pollution, exposing mammalian systems to a wide array of toxicants such as heavy metals, pesticides, and emerging micro- and nanoplastics. These pollutants exert their harmful effects through diverse cellular and molecular mechanisms such as oxidative stress, mitochondrial dysfunction, inflammation, apoptosis, and dysregulation of signalling pathways. Histopathological assessments have proven invaluable in revealing organ-specific structural and functional damage, making them essential endpoints in environmental toxicology. While advanced technologies like digital pathology, AI-based lesion detection, and integrative omics have significantly enhanced our ability to detect and characterise toxicological impacts. However, critical research gaps remain, including the lack of chronic, low-dose exposure models, standardised detection methods for micro- and nanoplastics in tissues, and insufficient mechanistic insight into emerging toxicants. Moreover, there is a notable scarcity of human epidemiological and histopathological data, highlighting the need for dedicated biobanks and tissue repositories. To effectively mitigate the health risks associated with environmental pollutants, future efforts must adopt a holistic, interdisciplinary approach, integrating histopathology, toxicology, environmental science, and public health, with priority given to developing harmonised protocols, enhancing mechanistic studies using high-resolution molecular tools, and translating scientific findings into actionable policy through robust regulatory toxicology and stakeholder engagement.

Conflict of interest

The authors declare no conflict of interest.

Abbreviations

AI	artificial intelligence
CdMT	cadmium-metallothionein
CKD	chronic kidney disease
DDT	dichlorodiphenyltrichloroethane
ETs	environmental toxicants
GCLC	glutamate-cysteine ligase catalytic subunit
HO-1	haem oxygenase-1
ICAM-1	intercellular adhesion molecule-1
KCs	Kupffer cells
MT	metallothionein
NADPH	nicotinamide adenine dinucleotide phosphate
NAFLD	non-alcoholic fatty liver disease
NASH	non-alcoholic steatohepatitis
NQO	quinine oxidoreductase
PAHs	polycyclic aromatic hydrocarbons
PM	particulate matter
POPs	persistent organic pollutants
PPAR	peroxisome proliferator-activated receptor
ROS	reactive oxygen species
UFPs	ultrafine particulates
VOCs	volatile organic compounds

Author details

Akinpelu Moronkeji[1*], Temidayo Daniel Adeniyi[2], Samuel Ayobami Fasogbon[3], Joshua Olayinka Ajala[4], Emmanuel Tolulope Adegoke[2], Comfort E. Williams[5], Abiodun Oyeleke[6], Charles Egede Ugwu[7], Olubunmi Esan[1], Bob-Manuel Chinonso Osuji[8] and Puritan Umeboro[9]

1 Department of Medical Laboratory Science, Faculty of Allied Health Sciences, University of Medical Sciences Ondo, Nigeria

2 Department of Medical Laboratory Science, Faculty of Basic Clinical Sciences, University of Ilorin, Ilorin, Kwara State, Nigeria

3 Department of Education, Medical Laboratory Science Council of Nigeria (MLSCN), Abuja City, FCT, Nigeria

4 Department of General Medicine, Kent and Canterbury Hospital, Canterbury, UK

5 Department of Pharmacology, New York Medical College, New York City, New York, USA

6 Department of Anatomy, Faculty of Basic Medical Sciences, Federal University Oye Ekiti, Ekiti State, Nigeria

7 Paul G. Allen School for Global Health, College of Veterinary Medicine, Washington State University, Pullman, WA, USA

8 School of Health and Life Sciences, Teesside University, Middlesbrough City, United Kingdom

9 Department of Medical Laboratory Sciences, Elizade University, Ilara-Mokin, Ondo State, Nigeria

*Address all correspondence to: amoronkeji@unimed.edu.ng

References

[1] Ibadi EA, Awad HK, Hussain LI. Environmental toxins and their organ-specific effects: A comprehensive review of human exposure and accumulation. Journal of Agricultural, Environmental and Veterinary Sciences (JAEVS). 2024;**8**(2):10-24

[2] Rebuzzini P, Fabozzi G, Cimadomo D, et al. Multi- and transgenerational effects of environmental toxicants on mammalian reproduction. Cells. 2022;**11**:1-24

[3] Moloudizargari M, Moradkhani F, Asghari N, et al. NLRP inflammasome as a key role player in the pathogenesis of environmental toxicants. Life Sciences. 2019;**231**:116585

[4] Matei E, Râpă M, Mateș IM, et al. Heavy metals in particulate matter—Trends and impacts on environment. Molecules. 2025;**30**:1-29

[5] Singh GK, Rai S, Jadon N. Major ambient air pollutants and toxicity exposure on human health and their respiratory system: A review. Journal of Environmental Management and Tourism. 2021;**12**:1774-1788

[6] Mack SM, Madl AK, Pinkerton KE. Respiratory health effects of exposure to ambient particulate matter and bioaerosols. Comprehensive Physiology. 2020;**10**:1-20

[7] Kaura S, Ding Y. Particulate matter with a diameter of 2.5 μm causes multiple pathological dysfunctions as presented by various biomarkers. Environmental Disease. 2019;**4**:57

[8] Shang M, Tang M, Xue Y. Neurodevelopmental toxicity induced by airborne particulate matter. Journal of Applied Toxicology. 2023;**43**:167-185

[9] Mitra S, Chakraborty AJ, Tareq AM, et al. Impact of heavy metals on the environment and human health: Novel therapeutic insights to counter the toxicity. Journal of King Saud University - Science. 2022;**34**:101865

[10] Adeniyi TD, Achukwu PU, Abubakar AA, et al. Heavy metals obtained from waterways induced neurodegeneration in the prefrontal cortex of Wistar rats. European Journal of Anatomy. 2019;**23**:65-76

[11] Phaenark C, Phankamolsil Y, Sawangproh W. Ecological and health implications of heavy metal bioaccumulation in Thai Fauna: A systematic review. Ecotoxicology and Environmental Safety. 2024;**285**:117086

[12] Jomova K, Alomar SY, Nepovimova E, et al. Heavy Metals: Toxicity and Human Health Effects. Berlin Heidelberg: Springer; 2025. DOI: 10.1007/s00204-024-03903-2

[13] Briffa J, Sinagra E, Blundell R. Heavy metal pollution in the environment and their toxicological effects on humans. Heliyon. 2020;**6**:e04691

[14] Angon PB, Islam MS, Shreejana KC, Das A, Anjum N, Poudel A, et al. Sources, effects and present perspectives of heavy metals contamination: Soil, plants and human food chain. Heliyon. 2024;**10**(7):e28357

[15] Das S, Sultana KW, Ndhlala AR, Mondal M, Chandra I. Heavy metal pollution in the environment and its impact on health: Exploring green Technology for Remediation.

Environmental Health Insights. 2023;**17**:11786302231201259. DOI: 10.1177/11786302231201259

[16] Abubakar US. Copper and lead as environmental pollutant and their elemental toxicity – A review. Scientific World Journal. 2024;**19**:342-346

[17] Zhu H, Tang X, Gu C, et al. Assessment of human exposure to cadmium and its nephrotoxicity in the Chinese population. Science of The Total Environment. 2024;**918**:170488

[18] Balali-Mood M, Naseri K, Tahergorabi Z, et al. Toxic mechanisms of five heavy metals: Mercury, lead, chromium, cadmium, and arsenic. Frontiers in Pharmacology. 2021;**12**:1-19

[19] Peana M, Pelucelli A, Medici S, et al. Metal toxicity and speciation: A review. Current Medicinal Chemistry. 2021;**28**:7190-7208

[20] Ahmad MF, Ahmad FA, Alsayegh AA, et al. Pesticides impacts on human health and the environment with their mechanisms of action and possible countermeasures. Heliyon. 2024;**10**:e29128

[21] Kaur R, Choudhary D, Bali S, et al. Pesticides: An alarming detrimental to health and environment. Science of The Total Environment. 2024;**915**:170113

[22] Zhou W, Li M, Achal V. A comprehensive review on environmental and human health impacts of chemical pesticide usage. Emerging Contaminants. 2025;**11**:100410

[23] Ray S, Shaju ST. Bioaccumulation of pesticides in fish resulting toxicities in humans through food chain and forensic aspects. Environmental Analysis, Health and Toxicology. 2023;**38**(2):e2023017. DOI: 10.5620/eaht.2023017

[24] Daraban GM, Hlihor RM, Suteu D. Pesticides vs. biopesticides: From pest management to toxicity and impacts on the environment and human health. Toxics. 2023;**11**(12):983. DOI: 10.3390/toxics11120983

[25] Mohammadi H, Ghassemi-Barghi N, Malakshah O, et al. Pyrethroid exposure and neurotoxicity: A mechanistic approach. Arhiv za Higijenu Rada i Toksikologiju. 2019;**70**:74-89

[26] Atere AD, Ajani OF, Moronkeji A, et al. Immunomodulatory response and serum level of neutrophil gelatinase associated lipocalin (NGAL) as a marker of acute kidney injury in Wistar rats exposed to pyrethroids. Journal of Cellular Biotechnology. 2021;7:99-109

[27] Atere AD, Moronkeji A, Moronkeji AI, et al. Serum levels of inflammatory biomarkers, glycaemic control indices and leptin receptors expression in adult male Wistar rats exposed to pyrethroids. Journal of Cellular Biotechnology. 2021;7:41-55

[28] Du Y, Nomura Y, Luo N, et al. Molecular determinants on the insect sodium channel for the specific action of type II pyrethroid insecticides. Toxicology and Applied Pharmacology. 2009;**234**:266-272

[29] Tsai YH, Lein PJ. Mechanisms of organophosphate neurotoxicity. Current Opinion in Toxicology. 2021;**26**:49-60

[30] Aroniadou-Anderjaska V, Figueiredo TH, de Araujo Furtado M, Pidoplichko VI, Braga MFM. Mechanisms of organophosphate toxicity and the role of acetylcholinesterase inhibition. Toxics. 2023;**11**(10):866. DOI: 10.3390/toxics11100866

[31] Ramírez-Mendoza AA, Mendoza-Magaña ML, Ramírez-Herrera MA,

Hernández-Nazara ZH, Domínguez-Rosales JA. Nitrooxidative stress and neuroinflammation caused by air pollutants are associated with the biological markers of neurodegenerative diseases. Antioxidants (Basel). 7 Mar 2024;**13**(3):326. DOI: 10.3390/antiox13030326

[32] Giesy JP, Solomon KR, Mackay D, et al. Evaluation of evidence that the organophosphorus insecticide chlorpyrifos is a potential persistent organic pollutant (POP) or persistent, bioaccumulative, and toxic (PBT). Environmental Sciences Europe. 2014;**26**:1-20

[33] Tasselli S, Marziali L, Roscioli C, Guzzella L. Legacy dichlorodiphenyltrichloroethane (DDT) pollution in a river ecosystem: Sediment contamination and bioaccumulation in benthic invertebrates. Sustainability. 2023;**15**(8):6493. DOI: 10.3390/su15086493

[34] Martyniuk CJ, Mehinto AC, Denslow ND. Organochlorine pesticides: Agrochemicals with potent endocrine-disrupting properties in fish. Molecular and Cellular Endocrinology. 2020;**507**:110764

[35] Soni D, Dass A, Yadav N, et al. Unveiling the invisible threat: A review of heavy metal exposure and its devastating health consequences. International Journal of Engineering Technology and Management Sciences. 2024;**8**:315-323

[36] Manisalidis I, Stavropoulou E, Stavropoulos A, et al. Environmental and health impacts of air pollution: A review. Frontiers in Public Health. 2020;**8**:1-13

[37] Ssedyabane F, Niyonzima N, Ngonzi J, Tusubira D, Ocan M, Akena D, et al. The diagnostic accuracy of serum microRNAs in detection of cervical cancer: A systematic review protocol. Diagnostic and Prognostic Research. 2023;**7**(1):4. DOI: 10.1186/s41512-023-00142-4

[38] Kaushal J, Khatri M, Arya SK. A treatise on organophosphate pesticide pollution: Current strategies and advancements in their environmental degradation and elimination. Ecotoxicology and Environmental Safety. 2021;**207**:111483

[39] Saha R, Dutta SM. Pesticides' mode of action on aquatic life. Toxicol Reports. 2024;**13**:101780

[40] Ram MA. Route of exposure and impact of pesticides pollution on human health and aquatic ecosystem. International Journal of Zoological Investigations. 2022;**08**:85-99

[41] Thakur M, Pathania D. Chapter 12 - Environmental fate of organic pollutants and effect on human health. In: Singh P, Kumar A, Borthakur A, editors. Abatement of Environmental Pollutants. Elsevier; 2020. pp. 245-262. DOI: 10.1016/B978-0-12-818095-2.00012-6

[42] Adeniyi T, Moronkeji A, Fikayomi A. Histological and biochemical evaluation of the protective potential of ascorbate and alpha-tocopherol against cypermethrin-induced toxicity. The Journal of Experimental Life Sciences. 2024;**14**:33-39

[43] Vergara-Gerónimo CA, León Del Río A, Rodríguez-Dorantes M, et al. Arsenic-protein interactions as a mechanism of arsenic toxicity. Toxicology and Applied Pharmacology. 2021;**431**:115738

[44] Speer RM, Zhou X, Volk LB, et al. Arsenic and cancer: Evidence and

mechanisms. Advances in Pharmacology. 2023;**96**:151-202

[45] Debnath T, Ghosh M, Lee YM, et al. Identification of phenolic constituents and antioxidant activity of *Aloe barbadensis* flower extracts. Food and Agricultural Immunology. 2018;**29**:27-38

[46] Chlubek M, Baranowska-Bosiacka I. Selected biochemical mechanisms of lead neurotoxicity. Pomeranian Journal of Life Sciences. 2023;**69**:33-39

[47] Zulaikhah ST, Wahyuwibowo J, Pratama AA. Mercury and its effect on human health: A review of the literature. International Journal of Public Health Science (IJPHS). 2020;**9**:103-114

[48] Azevedo LF, Karpova N, Rocha BA, Barbosa Junior F, Gobe GC, Hornos Carneiro MF. Evidence on neurotoxicity after intrauterine and childhood exposure to organomercurials. International Journal of Environmental Research and Public Health. 2023;**20**(2):1070. DOI: 10.3390/ijerph20021070

[49] Adeniyi T, Moronkeji A, Oluwatunase G, et al. Mercury-induced oxidative stress and neuropathologic changes in the prefrontal cortex of Wistar rats. Nigerian Journal of Neuroscience. 2024;**15**:97-104

[50] Moronkeji A, Adeniyi T, Olubunmi E, et al. Modulatory effects of *Aframomum melegueta* and *Rauvolfia vomitoria* in cadmium-induced renal toxicity in adult rats. Journal of Cellular Biotechnology. 2025;**11**(1):3-13. DOI: 10.1177/23523689251329719

[51] Moronkeji A, Temidayo A, Benita A, et al. Methanolic leaf extract of *Vernonia amygdalina* mitigates cadmium-induced oxidative stress in the liver and kidney of adult male Wistar rats. Egyptian Journal of Basic and Applied Sciences. 2024;**11**:469-478

[52] Zhang H, Reynolds M. Cadmium exposure in living organisms: A short review. Science of The Total Environment. 2019;**678**:761-767

[53] Genchi G, Sinicropi MS, Lauria G, Carocci A, Catalano A. The effects of cadmium toxicity. International Journal of Environmental Research and Public Health. 2020;**17**(11):3782. DOI: 10.3390/ijerph17113782

[54] Dewi R, Hamid ZA, Rajab NF, et al. Genetic, epigenetic, and lineage-directed mechanisms in benzene-induced malignancies and hematotoxicity targeting hematopoietic stem cells niche. Human & Experimental Toxicology. 2020;**39**:577-595

[55] Møller P, Folkmann JK, Forchhammer L, et al. Air pollution, oxidative damage to DNA, and carcinogenesis. Cancer Letters. 2008;**266**:84-97

[56] Moronkeji A, Akinbo FO. Genotoxic response and histological alterations in rat lungs exposed to gasoline generator exhaust. Sultan Qaboos University Journal for Science [SQUJS]. 2024;**29**:15-27

[57] Moronkeji A, Adeniyi TD, Atere AD. Oxidative stress response to gasoline generator exhaust emission in adult male Wistar rats. Environmental Analysis, Health and Toxicology. 2024;**39**:2-11

[58] Marchini T, Wolf D, Michel NA, et al. Acute exposure to air pollution particulate matter aggravates experimental myocardial infarction in mice by potentiating cytokine secretion from lung macrophages. Basic Research in Cardiology. 2016;**111**:1-14

[59] Jaiswal C, Singh AK. Particulate matter exposure and its consequences on hippocampal neurogenesis and cognitive function in experimental models. Environmental Pollution. 2024;**363**:125275

[60] Duque-Díaz E, Hurtado Giraldo H, Rocha-Muñoz LP, Coveñas R. Glyphosate, AMPA and glyphosate-based herbicide exposure leads to GFAP, PCNA and caspase-3 increased immunoreactive area on male offspring rat hypothalamus. European Journal of Histochemistry. 2022;**66**(4):3428. DOI: 10.4081/ejh.2022.3428

[61] Dowd FJ. Chapter 6—Cholinergic agonists and muscarinic receptor antagonists. In: Dowd FJ, Johnson BS, Mariotti AJBT-P, editors. Pharmacology and Therapeutics for Dentistry. 7th ed. Elsevier; 2017. pp. 82-97. DOI: 10.1016/B978-0-323-39307-2.00006-0

[62] Dzwilewski KLC, Schantz SL. Prenatal chemical exposures and child language development. Journal of Communication Disorders. 2015;**57**:41-65

[63] Banaee M. Perspective chapter: Exploring the toxicity effect of heavy metals on aquatic organisms – A comprehensive analysis. In: Heavy Metals in the Environment - Contamination, Risk, and Remediation. London, UK: IntechOpen; 2024. DOI: 10.5772/intechopen.1006890

[64] Bibi S, Naz S, Saeed S, et al. A review on histopathological alterations induced by heavy metals (Cd, Ni, Cr, Hg) in different fish species. Punjab University Journal of Zoology. 2021;**36**:81-89

[65] Jerrett M, Finkelstein MM, Brook JR, et al. A cohort study of traffic-related air pollution and mortality in Toronto, Ontario, Canada. Environmental Health Perspectives. 2009;**117**:772-777

[66] Knoblaugh SE, Hohl TM, La Perle KMD. Pathology principles and practices for analysis of animal models. ILAR Journal. 2018;**59**:40-50

[67] Aljehani Mohammad R, Alamri Fouad H, Elyas MEK, et al. The importance of histopathological evaluation in cancer diagnosis and treatment. International Journal of Health Sciences (Qassim). 2023;**7**:3614-3623

[68] Basaad A, Basurra S, Vakaj E, et al. A BERT-GNN approach for metastatic breast cancer prediction using histopathology reports. Diagnostics. 2024;**14**:1-20

[69] Oboma YI, Ekpenyong BO, Umar MS, et al. Histopathological, cytological and radiological correlations in allergy and public health concerns: A comprehensive review. Journal of Asthma and Allergy. 2024;**17**:1333-1354

[70] Gamde MS, Adeleye TM, Adisa JO. Review on histopathological techniques in cervical cancer screening. Asian Pacific Journal of Cancer Care. 2024;**9**:785-791

[71] Moronkeji A, Adeniyi T, Samuel A, Eze G, Akinbo F, Temidayo O, et al. Cervical lesion evaluation in females of reproductive age in Ondo town, Nigeria. Nigerian Medical Journal. 2025;**66**:407-419

[72] Liu Y, Xu J. High-resolution microscopy for imaging cancer pathobiology. Current Pathobiology Reports. 2019;**7**:85-96

[73] McGenity C, Clarke EL, Jennings C, et al. Artificial intelligence in digital pathology: A systematic review and meta-analysis of diagnostic test accuracy. npj Digital Medicine. 2024;**7**:6-9

[74] Neuberger J, Patel J, Caldwell H, et al. Guidelines on the use of liver biopsy in clinical practice from the British Society of Gastroenterology, the Royal College of Radiologists and the Royal College of pathology. Gut. 2020;**69**:1382-1403

[75] Wu B, Moeckel G. Application of digital pathology and machine learning in the liver, kidney and lung diseases. Journal of Pathology Informatics. 2023;**14**:100184

[76] Mehrvar S, Himmel LE, Babburi P, et al. Deep learning approaches and applications in toxicologic histopathology: Current status and future perspectives. Journal of Pathology Informatics. 2021;**12**:42

[77] Sanyal S, Crawford JA, Abraham JL. Overlooked role of histopathology in evaluations for occupational/environmental exposures. American Journal of Respiratory and Critical Care Medicine. 2020;**201**:1581

[78] Park SY, An KS, Lee B, et al. Establishment of particulate matter-induced lung injury model in mouse. Laboratory Animal Research. 2021;**37**:1-12

[79] Wang J, Li Y, Zhao P, et al. Exposure to air pollution exacerbates inflammation in rats with preexisting COPD. Mediators of Inflammation. 2020;**2020**(1):4260204. DOI: 10.1155/2020/4260204

[80] Van Pinxteren D, Brüggemann E, Gnauk T, Iinuma Y, Müller K, Nowak A, et al. Size-and time-resolved chemical particle characterization during CAREBeijing-2006: Different pollution regimes and diurnal profiles. Journal of Geophysical Research: Atmospheres. 2009;**114**(D2):D00G09. DOI: 10.1029/2008JD010890

[81] Srivastava D, Vu TV, Tong S, et al. Formation of secondary organic aerosols from anthropogenic precursors in laboratory studies. npj Climate and Atmospheric Science. 2022;**5**:22. DOI: 10.1038/s41612-022-00238-6

[82] Singh K, Tripathi D. Particulate matter and human health. In: Environmental Health. London, UK: IntechOpen; 2021. DOI: 10.5772/intechopen.100550

[83] Chang EM, Chao CC, Wang MT, et al. PM2.5 promotes pulmonary fibrosis by mitochondrial dysfunction. Environmental Toxicology. 2023;**38**:1905-1913

[84] Li Y, Lin B, Hao D, et al. Short-term PM2.5 exposure induces transient lung injury and repair. Journal of Hazardous Materials. 2023;**459**:132227

[85] Niu R, Cheng J, Sun J, Li F, Fang H, Lei R, et al. Alveolar type II cell damage and Nrf2-SOD1 pathway downregulation are involved in PM2. 5-induced lung injury in rats. International Journal of Environmental Research and Public Health. 2022;**19**(19):12893. DOI: 10.3390/ijerph191912893

[86] Xiong R, Jiang W, Li N, et al. PM2.5-induced lung injury is attenuated in macrophage-specific NLRP3 deficient mice. Ecotoxicology and Environmental Safety. 2021;**221**:112433

[87] Deng X, Rui W, Zhang F, et al. PM2.5 induces Nrf2-mediated defense mechanisms against oxidative stress by activating PIK3/AKT signaling pathway in human lung alveolar epithelial A549 cells. Cell Biology and Toxicology. 2013;**29**:143-157

[88] Shih C-H, Chen J-K, Kuo L-W, et al. Chronic pulmonary exposure to traffic-related fine particulate matter causes brain impairment in adult rats. Particle and Fibre Toxicology. 2018;**15**:1-17

[89] Gangwar RS, Bevan GH, Palanivel R, et al. Oxidative stress pathways of air pollution mediated toxicity: Recent insights. Redox Biology. 2020;**34**:101545

[90] Li R, Peng X, Wu Y, et al. Exposure to PM2.5 during pregnancy causes lung inflammation in the offspring: Mechanism of action of mogrosides. Ecotoxicology and Environmental Safety. 2021;**228**:112955

[91] Huang F, Wang P, Pan X, Wang Y, Ren S. Effects of short-term exposure to particulate matters on heart rate variability: A systematic review and meta-analysis based on controlled animal studies. Environmental Pollution. 2020;**256**:113306. DOI: 10.1016/j.envpol.2019.113306

[92] Ma N, Wei W, Fan X, Ci X. Farrerol attenuates cisplatin-induced nephrotoxicity by inhibiting the reactive oxygen species-mediated oxidation, inflammation, and apoptotic signaling pathways. Frontiers in Physiology. 2019;**10**:1419. DOI: 10.3389/fphys.2019.01419

[93] Ha JH, Lee BW, Yi DH, et al. Particulate matter-mediated oxidative stress induces airway inflammation and pulmonary dysfunction through TXNIP/NF-κB and modulation of the SIRT1-mediated p53 and TGF-β/Smad3 pathways in mice. Food and Chemical Toxicology. 2024;**183**:114201

[94] Kim YK, Jung JS, Lee SH, et al. Effects of antioxidants and Ca2+ in cisplatin-induced cell injury in rabbit renal cortical slices. Toxicology and Applied Pharmacology. 1997;**146**:261-269

[95] Slevin E, Baiocchi L, Wu N, et al. Kupffer cells: Inflammation pathways and cell-cell interactions in alcohol-associated liver disease. The American Journal of Pathology. 2020;**190**:2185-2193

[96] Xu GX, Wei S, Yu C, et al. Activation of Kupffer cells in NAFLD and NASH: Mechanisms and therapeutic interventions. Frontiers in Cell and Development Biology. 2023;**11**:1-13

[97] Arciello M, Gori M, Maggio R, et al. Environmental pollution: A tangible risk for NAFLD pathogenesis. International Journal of Molecular Sciences. 2013;**14**:22052-22066

[98] Zheng Z, Xu X, Zhang X, et al. Exposure to ambient particulate matter induces a NASH-like phenotype and impairs hepatic glucose metabolism in an animal model. Journal of Hepatology. 2013;**58**:148-154

[99] Tinkov AA, Aschner M, Santamaria A, et al. Dissecting the role of cadmium, lead, arsenic, and mercury in non-alcoholic fatty liver disease and non-alcoholic steatohepatitis. Environmental Research. 2023;**238**:117134

[100] Mentsiou Nikolaou E, Kalafati IP, Dedoussis GV. The interplay between endocrine-disrupting chemicals and the epigenome towards metabolic dysfunction-associated steatotic liver disease: A comprehensive review. Nutrients. 2024;**16**(8):1124. DOI: 10.3390/nu16081124

[101] Tovoli F, Stefanini B, Mandrioli D, et al. Exploring occupational toxicant exposures in patients with metabolic dysfunction-associated steatotic liver disease: A prospective pilot study. Digestive and Liver Disease. 2024;**56**:S53

[102] Jannetto PJ, Cowl CT. Elementary overview of heavy metals. Clinical Chemistry. 2023;**69**:336-349

[103] Rahman Z, Singh VP. The relative impact of toxic heavy metals (THMs) (arsenic (As), cadmium (Cd), chromium (Cr)(VI), mercury (Hg), and lead (Pb))

on the total environment: An overview. Environmental Monitoring Assessment. 2019;**191**(7):419. DOI: 10.1007/s10661-019-7528-7

[104] Jaishankar M, Tseten T, Anbalagan N, et al. Toxicity, mechanism and health effects of some heavy metals. Interdisciplinary Toxicology. 2014;**7**:60-72

[105] Katsarou A, Moustakas II, Pyrina I, et al. Metabolic inflammation as an instigator of fibrosis during nonalcoholic fatty liver disease. World Journal of Gastroenterology. 2020;**26**:1993-2011

[106] Satarug S, Vesey DA, Gobe GC. Current health risk assessment practice for dietary cadmium: Data from different countries. Food and Chemical Toxicology. 2017;**106**:430-445

[107] Rafati Rahimzadeh M, Rafati Rahimzadeh M, Kazemi SMA. Cadmium toxicity and treatment: An update. Caspian Journal of Internal Medicine. 2017;**2017**(8):135-145

[108] Klaassen CD, Liu J, Diwan BA. Metallothionein protection of cadmium toxicity. Toxicology and Applied Pharmacology. 2009;**238**:215-220

[109] Lin H-C, Hao W-M, Chu P-H. Cadmium and cardiovascular disease: An overview of pathophysiology, epidemiology, therapy, and predictive value. Revista Portuguesa de Cardiologia (English Edition). 2021;**40**:611-617

[110] Arab A, Mostafalou S. Neurotoxicity of pesticides in the context of CNS chronic diseases. International Journal of Environmental Health Research. 2022;**32**:2718-2755

[111] Elmorsy E, Al-Ghafari A, Al Doghaither H, Salama M, Carter WG. An investigation of the neurotoxic effects of Malathion, Chlorpyrifos, and Paraquat to different brain regions. Brain Sciences. 2022;**12**(8):975. DOI: 10.3390/brainsci12080975

[112] Naughton SX, Terry AV. Neurotoxicity in acute and repeated organophosphate exposure. Toxicology. 2018;**408**:101-112

[113] Tarafdar A, Pula G. The role of NADPH oxidases and oxidative stress in neurodegenerative disorders. International Journal of Molecular Sciences. 2018;**19**(12):3824. DOI: 10.3390/ijms19123824

[114] Cresto N, Forner-Piquer I, Baig A, et al. Pesticides at brain borders: Impact on the blood-brain barrier, neuroinflammation, and neurological risk trajectories. Chemosphere. 2023;**324**:138251

[115] Lafon PA, Wang Y, Arango-Lievano M, et al. Fungicide residues exposure and β-amyloid aggregation in a mouse model of Alzheimer's disease. Environmental Health Perspectives. 2020;**128**:1-20

[116] Hersh L, Rodgers D. Neprilysin and amyloid Beta peptide degradation. Current Alzheimer Research. 2008;**5**:225-231

[117] Tang BL. Neuropathological mechanisms associated with pesticides in Alzheimer's disease. Toxics. 2020;**8**:1-16

[118] Di DC, Chen CW, Chen YC, et al. Polystyrene microplastic particles: In vitro pulmonary toxicity assessment. Journal of Hazardous Materials. 2020;**385**:121575

[119] Aghaei Z, Mercer GV, Schneider CM, et al. Maternal exposure to polystyrene microplastics

alters placental metabolism in mice. Metabolomics. 2023;**19**:7-8

[120] Saleh SMM, Abdel-Zaher S, Mohamed MS, et al. Microplastics induced ileum damage: Morphological and immunohistochemical study. Microscopy Research and Technique. 2025;**88**:251-269

[121] Garcia MM, Romero AS, Merkley SD, Meyer-Hagen JL, Forbes C, Hayek EE, et al. In vivo tissue distribution of microplastics and systemic metabolomic alterations after gastrointestinal exposure. BioRxiv [Preprint]. 2023:2023.06.02.542598. DOI: 10.1101/2023.06.02.542598

[122] Ali SA, Rizk MZ, Hamed MA, et al. Assessment of titanium dioxide nanoparticles toxicity via oral exposure in mice: Effect of dose and particle size. Biomarkers. 2019;**24**:492-498

[123] Serrano QA, Le Garf S, Martin V, Colson SS, Chevalier N. Is physical activity an efficient strategy to control the adverse effects of persistent organic pollutants in the context of obesity? A narrative review. International Journal of Molecular Sciences. 2024;**25**(2):883. DOI: 10.3390/ijms25020883

[124] Fu Z, Bin XH, Elm J, et al. Formation of low-volatile products and unexpected high formaldehyde yield from the atmospheric oxidation of methylsiloxanes. Environmental Science & Technology. 2020;**54**:7136-7145

[125] World Health Organization. Ambient (outdoor) air pollution. In: Ambient (Outdoor) Air Pollution. Geneva, Switzerland: World Health Organization; 2022. Available from: https://www.who.int/news-room/fact-sheets/detail/ambient-(outdoor)-air-quality-and-health?gad_source=1&gclid=Cj0KCQjwvb-zBhCmARIsAAfUI2uht3D3H9sSC_f4cCZwKJkYFA1xGuiMGJc8xCmOuHgYhXC3yi7HDpgaAgJQEALw_wcB

[126] Guerrero-Limón G, Zappia J, Muller M. A realistic mixture of ubiquitous persistent organic pollutants affects bone and cartilage development in zebrafish by interaction with nuclear receptor signaling. PLoS One. 2024;**19**:1-24

[127] Landrigan PJ, Fuller R, Acosta NJR, et al. The lancet commission on pollution and health. Lancet. 2018;**391**:462-512

[128] Lodovici M, Bigagli E. Oxidative stress and air pollution exposure. Journal of Toxicology. 2011;**2011**:487074. DOI: 10.1155/2011/487074

[129] Tan W, Zhu H, Zhang N, et al. Characterization of the PM2.5 concentration in surgical smoke in different tissues during hemihepatectomy and protective measures. Environmental Toxicology and Pharmacology. 2019;**72**:103248

[130] Abadin H, Ashizawa A, Stevens YW, Llados F, Diamond G, Sage G, et al. Toxicological Profile for Lead. Atlanta (GA): Agency for Toxic Substances and Disease Registry (US); 2007

[131] Olawade DB, Wada OZ, Ige AO, et al. Artificial intelligence in environmental monitoring: Advancements, challenges, and future directions. Hygiene and Environmental Health Advances. 2024;**12**:100114

[132] Sies H, Jones DP. Reactive oxygen species (ROS) as pleiotropic physiological signalling agents. Nature Reviews. Molecular Cell Biology. 2020;**21**:363-383

[133] Sies H. On the history of oxidative stress: Concept and some aspects of

current development. Current Opinion in Toxicology. 2018;7:122-126

[134] Atkuri KR, Mantovani JJ, Herzenberg LA, et al. N-Acetylcysteine—A safe antidote for cysteine/glutathione deficiency. Current Opinion in Pharmacology. 2007;7:355-359

[135] Gurgueira SA, Lawrence J, Coull B, et al. Rapid increases in the steady-state concentration of reactive oxygen species in the lungs and heart after particulate air pollution inhalation. Environmental Health Perspectives. 2002;**110**:749-755

[136] Adeniyi TD, Akinpelu M, Omokehinde Oseni Akinlami FO, Alaga MMA. Evaluation of the combined extract of *Rauwolfia vomitoria* and *Aframomum melegueta* on the kidney and liver of adult male Wistar rats. Sokoto Journal of Medical Laboratory Science. 2024;**9**:203-212

[137] Zhang Z, Zhao L, Zhou X, et al. Role of inflammation, immunity, and oxidative stress in hypertension: New insights and potential therapeutic targets. Frontiers in Immunology. 2023;**13**:1-18

[138] Issa SY, Rahman SMA, Gaber YM, et al. Toxicological impact of Thiamethoxam on adult male rats: Histopathological, biochemical, and oxidative DNA damage assessment. Toxicol Reports. 2025;**14**:101983

[139] Song J, Shen Q, Shi J, et al. Changes in microbial community structure due to chronic trace element concentrations in different sizes of soil aggregates. Environmental Pollution. 2021;**268**:115933

[140] Zhao X, Wang S, Li X, et al. Cadmium exposure induces TNF-α-mediated necroptosis via FPR2/TGF-β/NF-κB pathway in swine myocardium. Toxicology. 2021;**453**:152733

[141] Cattaneo A, Campo L, Iodice S, et al. Environmental and biological monitoring of personal exposure to air pollutants of adult people living in a metropolitan area. Science of The Total Environment. 2021;**767**:144916

[142] Viegas S, Jeddi MZ, Hopf NB, et al. Biomonitoring as an underused exposure assessment tool in occupational safety and health context—Challenges and way forward. International Journal of Environmental Research and Public Health. 2020;**17**:1-20

[143] Wireman JR, Long GC. Communicating risk in diverse communities. Toxicology and Industrial Health. 2001;**17**:298-301

[144] Marchwińska-Wyrwał E, Teaf CM, Dziubanek G, et al. Risk assessment and risk communication in environmental health in Poland. European Journal of Public Health. 2012;**22**:742-744

[145] Shetty SS, Deepthi D, Harshitha S, Sonkusare S, Naik PB, Kumari SN, et al. Environmental pollutants and their effects on human health. Heliyon. 2023;**9**(9):e19496. DOI: 10.1016/j.heliyon.2023.e19496

[146] Lahr J, Kooistra L. Environmental risk mapping of pollutants: State of the art and communication aspects. Science of The Total Environment. 2010;**408**:3899-3907

[147] Marsili D, Pasetto R, Iavarone I. Environmental public health communication to engage stakeholders and foster social capacity in poorly involved communities living in industrial contaminated sites: The case study of Porto Torres (Italy). Frontiers in Communication. 2023;**8**:1217427. DOI: 10.3389/fcomm.2023.1217427

[148] Ward F, Lowther-Payne HJ, Halliday EC, et al. Engaging communities in addressing air quality: A scoping review. Environmental Health : A Global Access Science Source. 2022;**21**:1-18

[149] Collman GW. Community-based approaches to environmental health research around the globe. Reviews on Environmental Health. 2014;**29**:125-128

[150] Tan T, Junghans C, Varaden D. Empowering community health professionals for effective air pollution information communication. BMC Public Health. 2023;**23**:1-12

Chapter 2

Leachate Pollution Index: An Assessment and Treatment Strategy Designing Tool for Landfills

Rachna Jain and Dipanjali Majumdar

Abstract

Landfilling has been considered the most conventional, efficient, and cost-effective waste management technique for developed and developing nations. Traditionally, open dumping has been practiced in India for ages as a simple waste management solution which has now been gradually replaced by sanitary landfilling. Leachate, a seepage liquid percolated from both landfills, is a toxic cocktail of different industrial chemicals, heavy metals, micro and nanoparticle waste, and microbial metabolic products that make it a potential environmental threat. Leachate Pollution Index is a comprehensive tool for assessing and characterizing landfill leachate in terms of its pollution potential. The present study assesses the quality of leachate from both sanitary and open landfill in a typical urban environment under a tropical climate to understand the requisite rationale to identify potential treatment strategies using the leachate pollution Index as a tool. Samples were collected from an unlined open dump and a sanitary landfill site in West Bengal. Leachate pollution was assessed based on its physicochemical properties (BOD, COD, phenols, total coliforms, nitrogen, total dissolved solids (TDS), chlorides, and heavy metals) as per APHA standards. The cumulative leachate pollution potential due to organic, inorganic, and heavy metal components was reported in terms of the Leachate Pollution Index (LPI). LPI values for both sites were observed to be in the range of 12–24 units, significantly higher than the standard discharge limit (LPI ≤ 7.4), and hence they can be termed as a potential environmental threat that needs immediate attention before releasing to the environment.

Keywords: landfill, pollutant parameters, leachate pollution index, assessment, contamination

1. Introduction

Landfilling is considered to be the most convenient, economical, and effective waste management technique. Conventionally open dumping has been practiced worldwide, in which the entire trash has been dumped into an unlined piece of land. In landfill metabolic fluid, leachate seeps down from the heap and contaminates the whole environment, especially surface water, through which the pollutants seep down to the groundwater channel and, in between, contaminate the soil matrix. Leachate is a dark-colored toxic liquid comprising recalcitrant chemicals, POPs, pesticides, heavy metals, and microbial metabolic products [1]. There is no monitoring/control on the generation and spread of either leachate or other landfill emissions, and hence it becomes an open source for land, air, and water pollution [2].

1.1 Leachate pollution index (LPI)

Perilous discharge/recycling of wastewater results in terrestrial as well as aquatic pollution, resulting in adverse health impacts, poor soil quality, bad odor, etc. Discharge of contaminated water enhances the eutrophication process, which deteriorates dissolved oxygen content and hence affects aquatic flora and fauna [3–5]. Major fraction of this recycled water is used in irrigation, and other allied agricultural activities; heavily polluted discharge affects soil quality in terms of increased salinity, disturbed alkanity, bioaccumulation of industrial chemicals as well as heavy metals (Cu, Pb, Ag, Zn), etc. [6, 7]. Hence, monitoring discharged water is essential to determine the pollution threat.

LPI is a metric tool for the estimation of pollution potency of that particular landfill site, signifying the combination of toxicants being discharged into the environment, in order to design a suitable and effective treatment strategy to deal with this. The present study represents the comparative pollution potential of an open municipal solid waste dump and a lined engineered landfill site. LPI was calculated as per the waste fraction; for organics (LPI_{or}), inorganics (LPI_{in}), and heavy metals (LPI_{hm}), the cumulative LPI index of landfill sites was then observed by adding them together. The seasonal and temporal variations of sanitary landfill leachate on the basis of organic LPI fraction have been previously reported, and the order of potency was observed as $LPI\mathit{Summe}_{r}$ > LPI_{Winter} > $LPI_{Monsoon}$ [8]. Similarly, the microbial leachate treatment potential in terms of LPI reduction using organic and inorganic pollutant parameters was also reported [9]. However, the heavy metal profile is an important parameter that determines the toxicity potential of landfill sites. Hence, incorporating selected heavy metals is a key parameter for LPI calculation that helps in assessing the toxic characteristics of leachate along with its physicochemical pollution potential.

In lieu of this, the present study has been designed to evaluate the comprehensive comparative leachate pollution potential of an open landfill and a sanitary landfill. Leachate pollution potential was assessed individually as organic, inorganic, and heavy metal pollution and represented as cumulative LPI.

2. Materials and methods

All the chemicals used in the present study were of analytical grade > 99% purity.

2.1 Sampling site

2.1.1 Open landfill

Landfill leachate was collected from an adjacent open drain emerging from Dhapa Landfill, located at 22°32′09”N and 88°23′56″E. Dhapa is a well-known open heap of dump situated in the eastern fringes of Kolkata, West Bengal. It is spread in around 3 acres of land area and receives 2500 tons of waste per day. Dhapa is also known for ‘Garbage farming,’ and around 40% of green vegetables available in the local Kolkata markets is being supplied from here [10]. Dhapa open dump receives unsegregated waste. In the absence of any lining, the leachate formed from the mixed waste is uncontrolled that accumulates in small digs and leachate pools.

2.1.2 Sanitary landfill

A lined landfill site located in Baidyabati Municipality in West Bengal was chosen for this study. It is the first engineered landfill site in West Bengal, wherein segregated inert waste is dumped on an inclined surface and generated leachate seeps down and collected in a raw leachate pool [8, 9]. This raw leachate is further treated by the air stripping method in two consecutive aeration tanks and after sedimentation, this primarily treated leachate is discharged into nearby surface water bodies in **Figure 1**.

2.2 Sampling

Leachate samples were collected in winter 2021 from both sites by standard grab sampling method. From the sanitary landfill, two samples, before (raw; SLF-R) and after treatment (primary treated – SLF-PT), were collected. Samples were maintained and stored at 4°C in a refrigerator for analysis; for heavy metal estimation, samples were stored at low pH (pH 2–3). Microbial analysis was done within 6–8 hrs of sample collection.

2.3 *In situ* leachate characterization

Landfill leachate was characterized into three major waste components, that is, organic, inorganic, and heavy metals; the following pollutant parameters were observed under each category-

- *Organic part:* COD, BOD, total phenols, and total coliforms (TC)
- *Inorganic part:* pH, chloride, Total Dissolved Solids (TDS), Total Suspended Solids (TSS), Total Kjeldahl's Nitrogen (TKN)
- *Heavy metals:* Chromium (Cr), lead (Pb), arsenic (As), Zinc (Zn), Nickel (Ni), Copper (Cu), Iron (Fe)

All the parameters were analyzed using the standard APHA method [11].

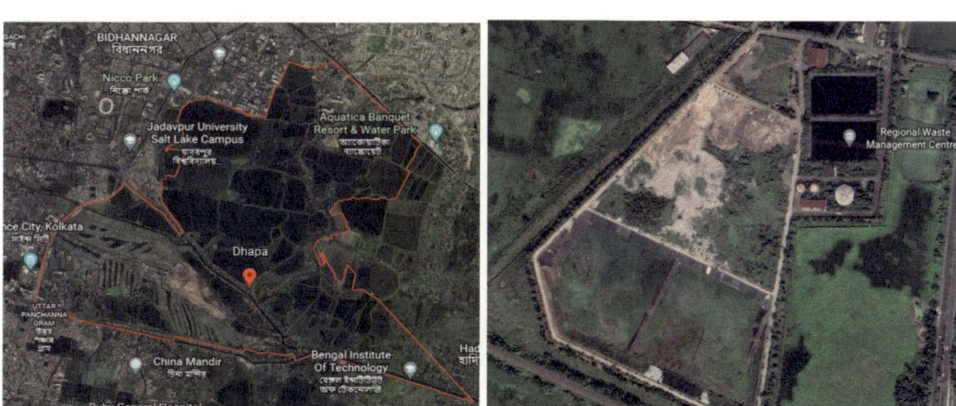

Figure 1.
Satellite view of Dhapa Open dumpsite and sanitary landfill site (Regional Waste Management Centre) Baidyabati.

2.4 Leachate pollution index (LPI)

LPI is a measure to determine the contamination potential of a landfill, which will further decide landfill condition and assess its remediation potential. On the basis of their status, landfills can be prioritized for management and remediation measures. The basic concept of LPI is an attempt to make an efficient system to compare the contamination potential of different landfills present in a given geographical area [12]. Eighteen different physicochemical parameters including organic, inorganic, and heavy metal fraction were used for the calculation of LPI, and their weight factors were ranked on a scale of 1 to 5 by the panelists [13]. The highest is given to heavy metal, followed by inorganic and organic pollutants. The order seems to follow the complexity in environmental reduction.

LPI of each fraction, organic, inorganic, and heavy metal waste, was calculated individually by the method described in our previous study [8]. Cumulative/overall LPI was then observed by adding them using the following equation:

$$\text{Overall } LPI = 0.232\text{LPI}_{or} + 0.257\, LPI_{in} + 0.511\, LPI_{hm}.$$

LPI_{or}, LPI of organic fraction; LPI_{in}, LPI of inorganic fraction; LPI_{hm}, LPI of heavy metal fraction.

Statistical analysis was done by using one-way ANOVA using SPSS 2021.

3. Results

3.1 Physicochemical characterization of leachate

Leachate samples collected from both open and sanitary landfills were observed to be highly polluted. Comparative analysis revealed that the pollution potential of open landfill is significantly higher (five to seven times) than that of both raw and primary treated leachate. The cumulative pollution overview depicted that TDS (52%), TSS (31%), and COD (8%) shared the maximum pollution load in an open landfill, whereas in a sanitary landfill, alkalinity and Total Kjeldahl's nitrogen (TKN) also contributed significantly, along with COD and TDS. Raw leachate possessed 41% TDS, 36% COD, 12% alkalinity, and 4% TKN as major pollutants; all the other organic, inorganic, and heavy metal fractions were present as micropollutants. Pollution parameters of primarily treated leachate were significantly less (13–81%) than both open dump and raw leachate, which clearly shows the efficiency of the air stripping method for leachate treatment, but still, the values were quite high, and hence this partially treated leachate cannot be considered safe for environmental discharge [9]. COD was observed to be the most prominent polluting factor, followed by TDS and alkalinity.

The BOD value of the raw and primary treated samples was found to be 285 and 214 mg/L, respectively, whereas in open landfill leachate, the parameter was five times higher. Similarly, COD varied between 4032 and 7715 mg/L. The organic waste fraction was majorly dominated by COD contamination, 70–96%, followed by BOD 4–13%. Open landfills also possessed 12% of the total coliform (TC) fraction. Total phenols shared a 0.019–0.004% fraction of the total pollution potential, with values in the range of 1.6–3.2 mg/L; although the percent share of TC and total phenols was less, they were still very much higher than the standard discharge limit and possessed a potential pollution threat.

In the inorganic fraction, TDS was a major contaminant in all three samples, that is, open dump (58%), raw leachate (65%), and primarily treated leachate (32%), with a concentration range of 1285–40,650 mg/L. TSS (34.5%) followed next in open landfill leachate, whereas in raw and primary treated leachate, alkanity followed TDS with 20 and 36% share, respectively. TKN concentration was observed to be 591–2781 mg/L and contributed 4, 7, and 14% share in open landfill, raw, and primary treated leachate, respectively. Chloride was also found to be significantly higher in primarily treated leachate samples; open landfill showed the least chloride content.

Among heavy metals, iron was the most polluting one; 30% was in open landfills, 59% was raw, and 63% was primarily treated leachate samples. Lead was the most dominant metal (36%) in the open landfill leachate, followed by 19% arsenic, whereas raw and primary treated leachate possessed 18 and 24% of nickel share. Copper also shared 2–3.19% while zinc was present in very low concentrations in all samples.

Variation in the pollution parameters in different classes, as evident, may be due to the diverse nature of the dumped waste [14, 15]. Open dump site receives comparatively more organic and municipal waste fractions and therefore, their BOD, COD, chloride, and TDS content are comparatively higher. On the other hand, in sanitary landfill sites, inert waste is dumped, and hence its organic parameters are significantly low (**Figure 2**) [16].

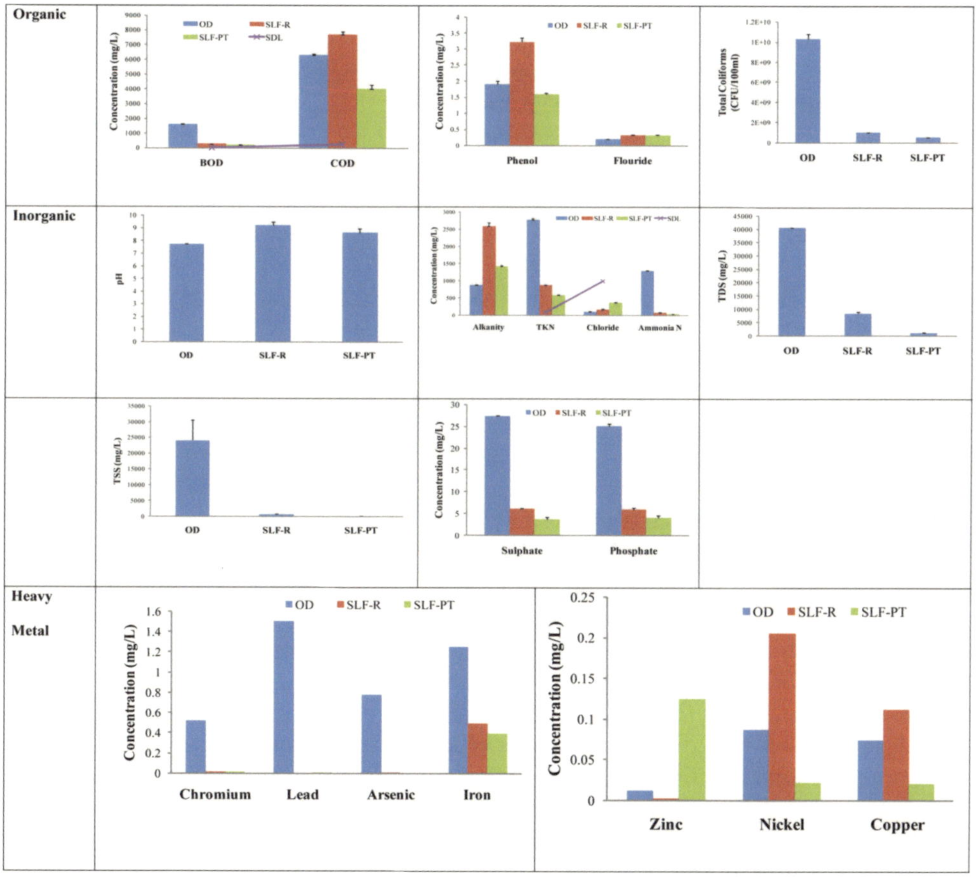

Figure 2.
Pollutant parameter distribution as per different fractions of waste.

Some prominent studies on leachate characterization in India and across the globe are listed below (**Table 1**).

Most of the studies reported above have focused only on major pollutant parameters, viz. BOD, COD, pH, nitrogen, and chlorides. In concurrence with our findings, studies done in India, Thailand, Indonesia, and Morocco have also reported high pollutant load in terms of BOD and COD from leachate samples collected from concentrated/open landfill sites. Dumping of unsegregated waste with compostable matter and high organic content may be the possible reason behind the high organic load in leachate. Whereas in sanitary landfills located in Malaysia, Virginia, and Beijing, the BOD/COD ratio was very low, corresponding to the higher inorganic fraction of dumped waste. The heavy metal content of the landfill leachate showed high variation as listed above. In India and Algeria, the heavy metal concentration was quite high compared to that of leachate collected from Ireland.

3.2 Leachate pollution index (LPI)

LPI of both landfill sites was calculated in terms of three fractions: organic, inorganic, and heavy metals. The fractional and cumulative LPI of both sites are described in **Table 2**.

LPI_{or} of open dump leachate was significantly higher, 11.03 LPI units, than sanitary leachate, 7.28, for primary treated and 8.26 LPI units for raw leachate as compared to standard 1.7968 (i.e., 23.2% of 7.4).

LPI_{in} of the open landfill is way higher than that of raw and primary treated sanitary leachate; 10.53, 3.37, and 2.36, respectively. Overall, the LPI of both sites was observed to be significantly higher than the standard 1.9 LPI units (25.7% of 7.4) with $R^2 \geq 0.9$. This huge difference may be due to the dumping of highly organic waste at open landfills; in contrast, only inert & non-recyclable waste is being discharged into the sanitary landfills, and therefore, the scope of generation of inorganic pollution is negated [8].

Heavy metal fraction of both open and sanitary leachate varied between 2.27 and 2.36 LPI units, which are lower than the standard value of 3.78 LPI units. But still, the concentration of analyzed toxic heavy metals, that is, As, Cu, Zn, Ni, Cr, Pb, and Fe, is significantly higher than their respective standard discharge limit.

3.2.1 Cumulative index: LPI

The cumulative LPI of the landfill site was calculated by the summation of all three factors as described by [13]. It was observed that the LPI of open landfill leachate was significantly higher (23.8 LPI units) than raw (14.4 LPI units) and primarily treated (12.01 LPI units) leachate samples. Aeration treatment seems to be an effective treatment strategy as both individual pollutant parameters, as well as LPI, pollution load have come down to a certain limit, but still, the values were quite high from the standards, that is, 7.4 LPI units for surface water discharge (**Figure 3**). Secondary treatment becomes quintessential in these circumstances to maintain environmental sustainability. LPI values in the present study are quite comparable with other reported Indian and International studies, as listed below. Variation in the LPI value may be attributed to different factors, viz. type of waste being dumped, frequency of dumping, the proportion of organic, inorganic as well heavy metal constituents; along with this, several environmental factors, temperature, humidity, tropical zone, rate of precipitation and capacity of landfill site also impacts the

Sl. No.	Location	Type of Landfill	Organic fraction (mg/L)		Inorganic fraction (mg/L)							Heavy Metals (ppb)						Reference
			BOD	COD	TDS	TSS	pH*	SO_4^{2-}	PO_4^{2-}	Ammonia Nitrogen/ T.N.	Cl^-	Pb	Cu	As	Ni	Zn	Ag	
1	Baydyabati, India	SF	214–285	4032–7716	1285–8604	744–2315	8.65–9.2	3.75–6	4.13–6	591–888	182–385	0.04–0.08	0.036	0.005	0.006–0.02	0.13–0.48	—	Present Study
2	Dhapa, India	CLL	1630	6317	40,649	24,140	7.76	27.4	25.13	2781	117.6	0.14	0.03	0.005	0.26	0.024	—	Present Study
3	Morocco	CLL	4707	13,743	NR	1264	7.8	NR	NR	4027	NR	NR	NR	NR	NR	NR	NR	[6]
4	Oman	CLL	2400–13,200	3600–33,600	5126–36,246	120–1270	8.2–8.6	36–417	16–68	562–4655	NR	BDL	1.83–6.41	BDL	BDL	BDL	NR	[17]
5	Brazil	CLL	NR	3542	NR	NR	NR	NR	NR	NR	3631	NR	NR	NR	NR	NR	NR	[18]
6		CLL	950	28,000	NR	NR	NR	NR	NR	3.50	NR	NR	NR	NR	NR	17.8	NR	[19]
7	Indonesia	CLL	3960	6280	NR	72.3	7.8	NR	NR	373.33	NR	NR	NR	NR	NR	NR	NR	[20]
8	Nonthaburi Landfill, Thailand	Semi-SF	760	3380	NR	NR	NR	NR	NR	1150	NR	NR	NR	NR	NR	1.35–1.6	NR	[21]
9	Varanasi, India	CLL	1335–3120	8300–12,000	2300–8322		8.8–9.1	NR	NR	NR	765–1221	ND	NR	ND	ND	ND	ND	[22]
10	Virginia, USA	SF	NR	4737	NR	NR	NR	NR	NR	1897	NR	NR	NR	NR	NR		NR	[23]
11	Brahmapuram, India	CLL	4250–5100	19,800–24,000	11,020–32,760	110–498	6.0–8.1	446–2597	184.88–268	1530–4000	2660–6700	NR	NR	NR	NR	NR	NR	[24]
12	Beijing, China	LL	105	2305	NR	NR	NR	NR	NR	1240	NR	NR	NR	NR	NR	NR	NR	[25]
13	Ireland	SF	33–984	190–7160	NR	NR	6.8–8.5	NR	NR	120–4027	160–2620	0.6–1047	0.003–2.423	11–412	10–661	10–7639	10–2187	[26]
14	Ludhiana, India	CLL	396–410	1335-2000	5300–6600	600–875	9.3–9.5	48–65	NR	NR	NR	TA	TA	TA	TA	TA	NR	[2]
15	India	CLL	1180–14,420	898–10,900	2740–7070	NR	8.2–8.6	345–456	NR	NR	285–368	NR	NR	NR	NR	NR	NR	[27]

Sl. No.	Location	Type of Landfill	Organic fraction (mg/L)		Inorganic fraction (mg/L)							Heavy Metals (ppb)						Reference
			BOD	COD	TDS	TSS	pH*	SO_4^{2-}	PO_4^{2-}	Ammonia Nitrogen/ T.N.	Cl^-	Pb	Cu	As	Ni	Zn	Ag	
16	Malaysia	CLL	326	2345	NR	NR	8.3	NR	NR	1568	NR	NR	NR	NR	NR	NR	NR	[28]
17	Malaysia	SF	83	935	NR	NR	7.7	NR	NR	540	NR	NR	NR	NR	NR	NR	NR	[28]
18	Algeria	CLL	900–980	3552–3792	NR	NR	8.27	2954–3056	48–58	55–85	4300–4500	3.49	0.39	NR	0.37	1.43	NR	[29]

CLL, concentrated landfill leachate; SF, sanitary landfills.

Table 1.
Review of reported studies on Leachate characterization across the globe.

DOI: http://dx.doi.org/10.5772/intechopen.1012094

Pollutant variable	Observed Concentration			Sub-Index Values			Weight Factors	Cumulative Pollution Ratings		
	OD	SLF-R	SLF-PT	OD	SLF-R	SLF-PT		OD	SLF-R	SLF-PT
COD	6317	7715	4032	65	70	60	0.267	17.36	18.69	16.02
BOD	1630	285	214	25	7	7	0.263	6.57	1.84	1.84
Phenol compounds	1.90	3.24	1.60	5	5	5	0.246	1.23	1.23	1.23
Coliforms	10,333	1025	560	100	70	55	0.224	22.4	15.68	12.32
LPI_o								47.56	37.44	31.41
								11.0339	*8.68631*	*7.287352*
pH	7.76	9.2	8.65	5	8	3	0.214	1.07	1.71	0.64
Chloride	117.65	183	385.04	5	5	5	0.187	0.93	0.93	0.93
TDS	40649.6	8603.67	1285.33	90	17	15	0.195	17.55	3.315	2.92
Total Kjeldahl's nitrogen	2781.05	888.257	591.13	8	28	18	0.206	1.65	5.77	3.71
Ammoniacal nitrogen	1305.11	92.6	46.67	100	7	5	0.198	19.8	1.39	0.99
LPI_i								41.003	13.12	9.2
								10.54	*3.38*	*2.36*
Chromium	0.008	0.02	0.024	5	5	8	0.125	0.625	0.625	1
Lead	0.14	0.082	0.044	6	7	5	0.123	0.738	0.861	0.615
Arsenic	0.005	0.005	0.000012	5	5	5	0.119	0.595	0.595	0.595
Zinc	0.024	0.131	0.484	5	7	8	0.11	0.55	0.77	0.88
Nickel	0.264	0.006	0.02	10	5	5	0.102	1.02	0.51	0.51
Copper	0.03	0.036	0.03	5	7	6	0.098	0.49	0.686	0.588
Iron	0.171	0.767	0.104	5	6	5	0.088	0.44	0.528	0.44
LPI_{hm}								4.458	4.575	4.628
								2.278	*2.338*	*2.365*
LPI Value								23.849	14.395	12.017

OD, open landfill leachate; SLF-R, raw sanitary landfill leachate; SLF, P.T., primary treated sanitary landfill leachate.

Table 2.
LPI of open and sanitary landfills.

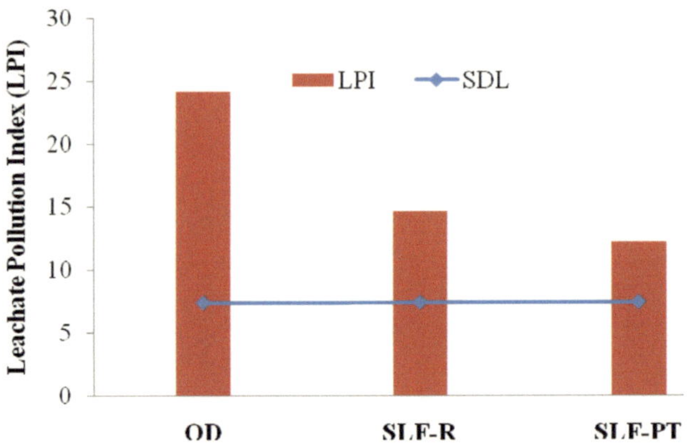

Figure 3.
Leachate Pollution Index in comparison to standard discharge limit.

leachate characteristics [12]. Seasonal variation also plays a major role in leachate characteristics, as depicted in our previous study [8]. The results of the study depict significantly higher LPI in the summer season than in winter and monsoon season. This is attributed to dilution of pollutants due to added surface run off and dew deposition, whereas in summer, the pollutants are concentrated due to excessive temperature, leading to a high vaporization rate. As compared to summer and monsoon, winters are meant to be a more stable season, reflecting the exact pollution scenario (**Table 3**).

Sl. No.	Location	Type of Landfill	LPI value	References
1	West Bengal, India	Active, Engineered	12.01–14.3	Present Study
2	West Bengal, India	Active, urban	23.8	Present Study
3	Multaqa landfill leachate, Oman	Active, urban	26	[17]
4	Barka landfill leachate, Oman	Active, urban	32.24	[17]
5	West Bengal, India	Active, Engineered	16–19.9	[9]
6	Hanoi, Vietnam	Urban, active	24.7	Hoai et al. [30]
7	Mutuail, Bangladesh	Active	19.81	Parvin & Tareq [31]
8	Ulu Maasop, Malaysia	Active, 36 years old, rural area	15.28	Hussein et al. [32]
9	Kampung Keru, Malaysia	Closed 29 years old urban area	13.89	Hussein et al. [32]
10	Ramma, India,	Rural, active	15.62	Mishra et al. [33]
11	Kerala, India	Active urban	31.99	Arunbabu et al. [34]
12	West Bengal, India	Active, urban	28.9	[35]
13	Mohali, India	Urban	27	Rana et al. [36]
14	Warri, Nigeria	Urban, active	6.37–7.43	Godwin & Oghenekohwiroro [37]

Table 3.
Reported LPI index of different landfill sites as compared to the present study.

3.3 LPI: A potential tool for identification of suitable secondary leachate treatment strategy

In addition to the assessment of the pollution potential of a particular landfill site, LPI can also be used as a tool for identifying appropriate treatment strategies. Based on LPI fractionation, it is evident that organic, inorganic, and heavy metal fractions share 23.2, 25.7, and 51.1% of the cumulative LPI of the particular site. Therefore, the individual LPI value of each fraction should not exceed 1.8 (LPI_{or}), 1.9 (LPI_{in}), and 3.78 (LPI_{hm}) for safe and sustainable water discharge. Based on this, a suitable treatment strategy can be designed, that is, if

- LPI_{or} is >1.8 – Biological treatment.
- LPI_{in} is >1.9 – Physicochemical and Advance oxidation.
- LPI_{hm} is >3.78 – Adsorption, Oxidation, etc.

But in general, all three factors are aligned with each other, and hence, a combined treatment strategy is always effective than standalone ones. Also, the applied treatment technology depends on the ultimate use of treated water; that is, if the ultimate use is drinking, then advanced oxidation and nanoparticle-based methods can be used, but if the treated water is meant for surface discharge, then high-end technologies can be avoided. Different researchers have reported physicochemical (stripped air, coagulation, flocculation), biological (using bacteria, fungi, algae, plants, etc.), and advanced oxidation methods (ionization, Fenton, RO) for leachate treatment [38–43]. The present study reports significantly higher organic (LPI 7.2–11.03) and inorganic (LPI 2.36–10.54) pollution loads; hence, combined physicochemical and biological treatment methods would be appropriate for treatment purposes. However, standalone physicochemical methods are quite expensive, generate a lot of sludge, and are not suitable for large-scale implementation; hence, a combined strategy can be a sustainable solution [16].

Irrespective of the efficiency of the method applied, it is mandatory to monitor the treatment process carefully so that the ecological balance is not disturbed. Most wastewater treatment technologies lead water up to surface water standards, and it is mainly used for irrigation and domestic use, as detailed below.

Based on the leachate containment potential, the following treatment strategies may be recommended for implementation at engineered landfill sites (**Figure 4**).

3.4 Wastewater use/disposal

Apart from toxic chemicals, pesticide residues and other recalcitrant chemicals, wastewater is also a huge source of phosphates, nitrates, and other micronutrients required for soil fertility, therefore treated wastewater can be easily applied on soils for agricultural use, which will in turn, reduce 25–50% of fertilizer use and increase the crop productivity by 15–27% as compared to normal water irrigation. In the small cities of Gujrat, the selling of sewage/wastewater is a regular income generation practice. In peri-urban areas, wastewater irrigation practices increase vegetable and other perishable production, that is, fodder, etc., by four times in a single piece of land [44]. Individual data and reports on leachate disposal are not available, and hence, consolidated wastewater generation and disposal strategies are explained below.

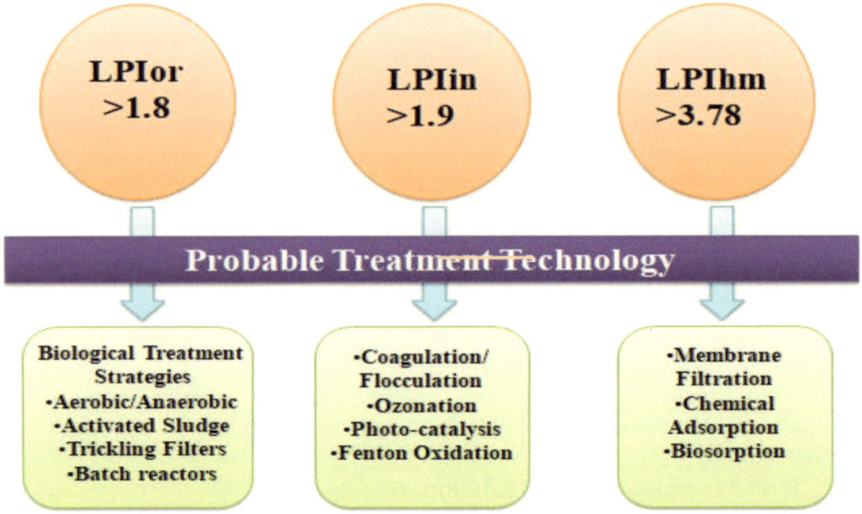

Figure 4.
Possible Leachate treatment strategies.

Wastewater-based irrigation is being done all around the country; major production and places are listed below (**Table 4**).

3.5 Hurdles in safe water discharge: Status and need for the knowledge and skills on the safe use of wastewater

- The high salinity of wastewater decreases soil productivity. Therefore, only tolerant plants can be grown in those places [45].
- Excessive release of industrial effluent results in toxin accumulation that promotes the overgrowth of weeds, algae, and cyanobacteria and deteriorates groundwater and downstream water quality.
- Wastewater is a rich source of plant nutrients; therefore, excess fertilizers should be applied accordingly.

Sl. No	Name of the Crop	Place
1	Cereals (Paddy, Wheat)	Hyderabad, Ahmedabad, Kanpur
2	Vegetables (Cucurbits, eggplant, okra, amaranths, mint, and coriander in the summers; Spinach, mustard, cauliflower, and cabbage in the winters)	New Delhi, Hyderabad
3	Flowers (roses, marigold, and Jasmine)	Kanpur & Hyderabad
4	Avenue trees and parks	Hyderabad
5	Aquaculture	East Kolkata
6	Agroforestry (sapota, guava, coconut, mango, arecanut, teak, neem, banana, Ramphal, curry leaf, pomegranate, lemon, galimara, mulberry, etc.)	Hubli-Dharwad in Karnataka

Table 4.
Reported literature on wastewater-based irrigation.

- Regular soil testing is essential to understand nutrient requirements.
- For certain crops, especially fodder crops, irrigation must be stopped before 1–2 weeks of harvesting so that the pollutants cannot accumulate in the crops.
- On heavily contaminated lands, non-food crops with high economic value, like sisal, mahogany, Eucalyptus, poplar, bamboo, neem (*Azadirachta indica*), shisha (*Dalbergia sissoo*), etc., can be grown to develop a green belt around the city. These plants accumulate pollutants in their root, and hence the groundwater is not much polluted. Biochemical oxygen demand removal efficiency of tree plantations has also been observed to be 80.0–94.3% [46].
- A selective cultivation approach can be used to accumulate maximum pollutants from the wastewater into the non-edible parts. It should be promoted in public parks, golf courses, green belts, and tree plantations.
- Efficient strains of microbes for wastewater remediation should be searched out and applied at the field scale.
- Increased funding may be provided for research to design efficient, cost-effective, and sustainable natural wastewater treatment systems that conserve nutrients while effectively removing pathogens and other pollutants.
- Wastewater should be appropriately diluted so that the toxin remains below the lethal dose and does not affect crop productivity.

4. Conclusion

Leachate is a potential source of water pollution and is a hidden threat to environmental sustainability. Hence, regular monitoring of landfill leachate is necessary to keep an eye on the possibility of creating pollution in the nearby surface as well as groundwater bodies. Leachate samples analyzed in the present study were found to be heavily contaminated, as depicted by significantly higher values of all the organic and inorganic pollutant parameters. Therefore, direct discharge of this effluent from both open dumps and sanitary landfill sites is not feasible, and the application of an appropriate treatment strategy is the need of the hour.

Regular quality checks of the discharge effluent will help in designing suitable treatment strategies for better management of waste in the landfill and ultimately result in a clean and green environment.

Acknowledgements

The authors gratefully acknowledge the guidance and support of the Director, CSIR-NEERI, and the Chair, CSIR-NEERI, Kolkata Zonal Center. The authors also acknowledge the mentorship of Dr. Saravana Devi Sivanesan, Chief Scientist, CSIR-NEERI, Nagpur, for her constant support. The KRC (Knowledge Resource Center of CSIR-National Environmental Engineering Research Institute) number for the manuscript is CSIR-NEERI/KRC/2025//SEP/KZC/1.

Author details

Rachna Jain* and Dipanjali Majumdar
Kolkata Zonal Centre, i-8, Sector-C, CSIR-National Environmental Engineering Research Institute (NEERI), Kolkata, India

*Address all correspondence to: rachna11587@gmail.com and ra_jain@neeri.res.in

References

[1] Ishak AR, Mohamad S, Soo TK, Hamid FS. Leachate and surface water characterization and heavy metal health risk on cockles in Kuala Selangor. Procedia - Social and Behavioral Sciences. 2016;**222**:263-271

[2] Bhalla B, Saini MS, Jha MK. Characterization of leachate from municipal solid waste (MSW) landfilling sites of Ludhiana, India: A comparative study. International Journal of Engineering Research and Applications. 2012;**2**(6):732-745

[3] Maiti SK, De S, Hazra T, Debsarkar A, Dutta A. Characterization of leachate and its impact on surface and groundwater quality of a closed dumpsitelandfill – A case study at Dhapa, Kolkata, India. Procedia Environmental Sciences. 2016;**35**:391-399

[4] Mor S, Negi P, Khaiwal R. Assessment of groundwater pollution by landfills in India using leachate pollution index and estimation of error. Environmental Nanotechnology, Monitoring and Management. 2018;**10**:467-476

[5] Salami L, Fadayini O, Patinvoh RJ, Koleola O. Evaluation of leachate contamination potential of Lagos dumpsite landfills using leachate pollution index. British Journal of Applied Science & Technology. 2015;**5**(1):48-59

[6] Rhoualem F, Hadiri HE, Oukour N, Taouil H, Arouyaa K, Ahmed SI. Physico-chemical characterization of leachate from the Moulay Abdallah technical landfill center (Morocco). Ecological Engineering. 2022;**23**(8):241-248

[7] Sriram S, Mandla VR, Sudha CM, Subba Rao SSV, Nagaveni C, Vani V, et al. Study of leachate characterization in landfill by municipal solid waste. Research Journal of Pharmacy and Technology. 2017;**10**(2):385-390

[8] Jain R, Majumdar D, Mondal R. In spatial modeling and assessment of environmental contaminants. In: Environmental Challenges and Solutions. UK: Springer; 2021. pp. 29-53

[9] Jain R, Majumdar D, Devi S. Microbial treatment of raw and primary treated sanitary landfill leachate by indigenous strain *Brevibacillus agri*. Applied Biochemistry and Biotechnology. 2022;**195**(4):2317-2331. DOI: 10.1007/s12010-022-04056-7

[10] De S, Maiti SK, Hazra T, Debsarkar A, Dutta A. Appraisal of seasonal variation of groundwater quality near an uncontrolled municipal solid waste landfill in Kolkata, India. Glob Nest Journal. 2017;**19**(3):367-376

[11] APHA. Standard Methods for Examination of Water and Wastewater. 22nd ed. Washington D.C.: APHA; 2012

[12] Umar M, Aziz HA, Yusoff MS. Variability of parameters involved in leachate pollution index and determination of LPI from four landfills in Malaysia. International Journal of Chemical Engineering. 2010;**2010**:747953

[13] Kumar D, Alappat BJ. Evaluating leachate contamination potential of landfill sites using leachate pollution index. Clean Technologies and Environmental Policy. 2005;**7**(3):190-197

[14] Adhikari B, Dahal R, Khanal N. A review of factors affecting the composition of municipal solid waste landfill leachate. International Journal

of Engineering Science and Innovative Technology. 2014;**3**:273-281

[15] Chofqi A, Younsi A, Lhadi EK, Mania J, Mudry J, Veron A. Environmental impact of an urban landfill on a coastal aquifer (El Jadida, Morocco). Journal of the African Earth Sciences. 2004;**39**(3-5):509-516

[16] Jain R, Majumdar D, Chatterjee S. Heavy Metals and Antibiotic Sensitivity Indexing of four Indigenous Landfill Strains Bulletin of Environmental Contamination and Toxicology. 2024,**113**(1):3. DOI: 10.1007/s00128-024-03903-z

[17] Siddiqi SA, Mamun AA, Sana A, Baawain MS, Choudhury RM. Characterization and pollution potential of leachate from urban landfills during dry and wet periods in arid regions. Water Supply. 2021;**22**(3):3462. DOI: 10.2166/ws, 392

[18] Destro GE, Junior Braga SS, Yasmin TS, Alaor AA, Chaves AR, Forti JC. Characterization of leachate produced by a landfill and its influence on a sewage treatment plant. Environmental Quality Management. 2020;**30**(1):15-23

[19] Ren X, Liu D, Chen W, Jiang G, Wu J, Song K. Investigation of the characteristics of concentrated leachate from six municipal solid waste incineration power plants in China. RSC Advances. 2018;**8**:13159. DOI: 10.1039/c7ra13259j

[20] Noerfitriyani E, Hartono DM, Moersidik SS, Gusniani I. Leachate characterization and performance evaluation of leachate treatment plant in Cipayung landfill, Indonesia. IOP Conference Series: Earth and Environmental Sciences. 2018;**106**:012086. DOI: 10.1088/1755 1315/106/1/012086

[21] Xaypanya P, Takemura J, Chiemchaisri C, Seingheng H, Tanchuling MAN. Characterization of landfill leachates and sediments in major cities of Indochina peninsular countries – Heavy metal partitioning in municipal solid waste leachate. Environments. 2018;**5**:65. DOI: 10.3390/environments 5060065

[22] Mishra S, Tiwary D, Ohri A. Leachate characterisation and evaluation of leachate pollution potential of urban municipal landfill sites. International Journal of Environment and Waste Management. 2018;**21**:217

[23] Iskandar SM, Novak JT, Brazil B, He Z. Simultaneous energy generation and U.V. Quencher removal from landfill leachate using a microbial fuel cell. Environmental Science and Pollution Research. 2017;**24**:26040-26048. DOI: 10.1007/ s11356-017-0231-8

[24] Nivya TK, Minimol Pieus T. Comparison of photo ElectroFenton process (PEF) and combination of PEF process and membrane bioreactor in the treatment of landfill leachate. Procedia Technology. 2016;**24**:224-231

[25] Wang Z, Peng Y, Miao L, Cao T, Zhang F, Wang S, et al. Continuous-flow combined process of nitritation and ANAMMOX for treatment of landfill leachate. Bioresource Technology. 2016;**214**:514-519. DOI: 10.1016/j.biortech

[26] Brennan RB, Healy MG, Morrison L, Hynes S, Norton D, Clifford E. Management of landfill leachate: The legacy of European Union directives. Journal of Waste Management. 2015;**55**:355-363

[27] Reddy SP, Nandini N. Leachate characterization and assessment of groundwater pollution near municipal solid waste landfill site. Nature,

Environment and Pollution Technology. 2011;**10**(3):415-418

[28] Aziz SA, Aziz S, Aziz HA, Yusoff MS, Bashir Umar M. Leachate characterization in semi-aerobic and anaerobic sanitary landfills: A comparative study. Journal of Environmental Management. 2010;**91**(12):2608-2614

[29] Salem Z, Hamouri K, Djemaa R, Allia K. Evaluation of landfill leachate pollution and treatment. Desalination. 2008;**220**:108-114

[30] Hoai ST, Nguyen LH, Thi VNT, Nguyen HG, Kawamoto K. Characterizing seasonal variation in landfill leachate using leachate pollution index (LPI) at Nam son solid waste landfill in Hanoi, Vietnam. Environments. 2021;**8**(3):17

[31] Parvin F, Tareq SM. Impact of landfill leachate contamination on surface and groundwater of Bangladesh: A systematic review and possible public health risks assessment. Applied Water Science. 2021;**11**(6):100

[32] Hussein M, Yoneda K, Zaki ZM, Othman NA, Amir A. Leachate characterizations and pollution indices of active and closed unlined landfills in Malaysia. Environmental Nanotechnology, Monitoring and Management. 2019;**12**:100232

[33] Mishra S, Tiwary D, Ohri A, Agnihotri AK. Impact of municipal solid waste landfill leachate on groundwater quality in Varanasi, India. Groundwater for Sustainable Development. 2019;**9**:100230

[34] Arunbabu V, Indu KS, Ramasamy EV. Leachate pollution index as an effective tool in determining the phytotoxicity of municipal solid waste leachate. Journal of Waste Management. 2017;**68**:329-336

[35] Naveen BP, Mahapatra MD, Sitharam TG, Sivapullaiah PV, Ramachandra TV. Physico-chemical and biological characterization of urban municipal landfill leachate. Environmental Pollution. 2016;**220**:1-12

[36] Rana R, Ganguly R, Gupta AK. Indexing method for assessment of pollution potential of leachate from non-engineered landfill sites and its effect on ground water quality. Environmental Monitoring and Assessment. 2017;**190**(1):46

[37] Godwin A, Oghenekohwiroro E. Leachate characterization and leachate pollution index from landfill dump sites in Warri Metropolis, Nigeria. International Letters of Natural Sciences. 2016;**57**:41-48

[38] Cui YH, Xue WJ, Yang SQ, Tu JL, Guo XL, Liu ZQ. Electrochemical/peroxydisulfate/Fe3þ treatment of landfill leachate nanofiltration concentrate after ultrafiltration. Chemical Engineering Journal. 2018;**353**:208-217. DOI: 10.1016/j.cej.2018.07.101

[39] Dabaghian Z, Peyravi M, Jahanshahi M, Rad AS. Potential of advanced nano-structured membranes for landfill leachate treatment: A review. Chem Bio Eng Reviews. 2019;**5**:1-20. DOI: 10.1002/cben.201600020

[40] de Oliveira MS, da Silva LF, Barbosa AD, Romualdo L, Sadoyama G, Andrade LS. Landfill leachate treatment by combining coagulation and advanced electrochemical oxidation techniques. Chem Electro Chem. 2019;**6**:1427-1433. DOI: 10.1002/celc.201801677

[41] Dolar D, Košutic K, Strmecky T. Hybrid processes for treatment of landfill

leachate: Coagulation/UF/NF-RO and adsorption/UF/NF-RO. Separation and Purification Technology. 2016;**168**:39-46. DOI: 10.1016/j.seppur.2016.05.016

[42] Er XY, Seow TW, Lim CK, Ibrahim Z, Mat Sarip SH. Biological treatment of closed landfill leachate treatment by using *Brevibacillus panacihumi* strain ZB1. IOP Conference Series: Earth Environmental Sciences. 2019;**140**:012012. DOI: 10.1088/1755-1315/140/1/012012

[43] Erabee IK, Ahsan A, Jose B, Aziz MMA, Ng AWM, Idrus S, et al. Adsorptive treatment of landfill leachate using activated carbon modified with three different methods. KSCE Journal of Civil Engineering. 2018;**22**(4):1083-1095. DOI: 10.1007/s12205-017-1430-z

[44] Minhas PS, Samra JS. Wastewater use in peri-urban agriculture: Impacts and opportunities. Bulletin No. 2. 2004;**6**:100224

[45] Banik E, Singh R. Analysis of waste water treatment in India. Research Explorer-A Blind Review & Refereed Quarterly International Journal. 2020;**III**(27):40-46

[46] Thawale PR, Juwarkar AA, Singh SK. Resource conservation through land treatment of municipal wastewater. Current Science. 2006;**90**:704-711

Chapter 3

The Impact of Heavy Metals on Pancreatic β-Cell Function: Mechanisms and Implications for Development of Diabetes Mellitus

Tugba Kose

Abstract

Environmental exposure to heavy metals is an increasingly recognized risk factor in the development of metabolic disorders, including diabetes mellitus (DM). Pancreatic β-cells are particularly vulnerable to oxidative and functional damage induced by toxicants such as cadmium (Cd), arsenic (As), lead (Pb), and manganese (Mn); however, the mechanisms of toxicity remain inadequately defined. This study aimed to evaluate the cytotoxic, oxidative, and functional effects of $CdCl_2$, $NaAsO_2$, $MnCl_2$, and $PbCl_2$ on insulin-secreting MIN6 and INS-1 pancreatic β-cell lines. Cells were exposed to different concentrations of heavy metals for 24 h. Cell viability was assessed using the 3-(4,5-dimethylthiazol-2-yl)-2,5-diphenyl tetrazolium bromide (MTT) assay, while intracellular reactive oxygen species (ROS) and lipid peroxidation (measured as malondialdehyde, MDA), were quantified to determine oxidative stress. Glucose-stimulated insulin secretion (GSIS) was evaluated using a high glucose challenge and ELISA-based insulin quantification. Exposure to 2 μM $CdCl_2$ and $NaAsO_2$, and 5 μM $MnCl_2$ and $PbCl_2$, significantly reduced cell viability and insulin secretion in both cell lines. These treatments also induced a marked increase in ROS generation and malondialdehyde (MDA) levels, indicating enhanced oxidative stress and lipid peroxidation. Cd, As, Pb, and Mn exert dose-dependent cytotoxic effects on pancreatic β-cells by impairing viability, disrupting insulin secretion, and inducing oxidative stress. These findings support the hypothesis that chronic exposure to heavy metals contributes to β-cell dysfunction, and may play a role in diabetes pathogenesis. Gaining insight into these mechanisms is essential for guiding environmental health policies and creating targeted intervention strategies.

Keywords: heavy metals, pancreatic cell damage, diabetes mellitus, oxidative stress, environmental health

1. Introduction

Exposure to environmental pollutants is often underestimated; however, significant risk factors in the development and progression of various chronic diseases [1]. Despite increasing awareness, the role of these pollutants, particularly toxic heavy metals, in metabolic disorders such as diabetes mellitus (DM) remains insufficiently explored. Epidemiological and experimental studies have drawn growing attention to the association between environmental toxicants and the global rise in diabetes prevalence [1, 2].

DM is a multifaceted metabolic disorder characterized by chronic hyperglycemia, resulting from impaired insulin resistance, insulin secretion, or a combination of both. It exists primarily in two forms: Type I (insulin-dependent) and type II (non-insulin-dependent) [3]. Emerging evidence suggests that exposure to environmental pollutants can overload pancreatic β-cells, induce cellular stress, and impair their functional capacity. In addition to promoting insulin resistance and disrupting glucose metabolism, these pollutants can directly damage pancreatic islets, contributing to diabetes pathogenesis [2]. Given the rising environmental burden of disease, there is a pressing need for comprehensive research into the mechanisms by which environmental contaminants contribute to diabetes.

Cadmium (Cd) is among the most harmful toxic metal pollutants, known for its ability to bioaccumulate over time and exert toxic effects on multiple organ systems, including the kidneys, bones, and pancreas [4–6]. Cd is commonly used in industrial processes, such as battery production, pigments, and plastic manufacturing, and is ranked seventh on the U.S. Agency for Toxic Substances and Disease Registry's Substance Priority List [7]. In nonoccupational environments, cadmium (Cd) exposure primarily happens through contaminated food, water, and tobacco smoke. Prolonged Cd exposure has been associated with nephrotoxicity, cancer, bone damage, and metabolic disturbances, including hyperglycemia and hypoinsulinemia [5, 8].

Arsenic (As), another widespread environmental pollutant, is commonly found in groundwater and industrial waste [9]. Chronic arsenic exposure is associated with oxidative stress, inflammation, and DNA damage, all of which can impair pancreatic β-cell function [10]. Epidemiological data link arsenic exposure to increased insulin resistance, glucose intolerance, and diabetes risk, particularly in populations with high levels of arsenic in drinking water [9, 10].

Lead (Pb), although now less commonly used in industrial materials due to regulatory controls, remains an environmental hazard due to its persistence in soil and water [11]. Pb exposure has been shown to alter calcium signaling pathways, essential for insulin granule exocytosis. *In vitro*, $PbCl_2$ has been reported to reduce insulin secretion and increase lipid peroxidation in INS-1 cells [12]. Moreover, Pb exposure enhances ROS production, promoting oxidative DNA damage and impairing β-cell function, as shown in studies using both β-cell lines and isolated islets [13, 14].

Manganese (Mn), though essential in small amounts for enzymatic and metabolic functions, can be neurotoxic and metabolically disruptive at high levels [15]. Excess Mn has been linked to impaired insulin signaling, mitochondrial dysfunction and β-cell apoptosis [16]. *In vitro* investigations using MIN6 cells revealed that high Mn concentrations cause a significant increase in ROS and a reduction in insulin secretion [14, 17]. Additionally, studies have shown that Mn disrupts the antioxidant defense system, including enzymes such as superoxide dismutase (SOD) and catalase, making β-cells more susceptible to oxidative injury [16, 18].

To investigate the cellular and molecular mechanisms underlying heavy metal-induced pancreatic damage, *in vitro* models such as INS-1 (rat insulinoma) and MIN6 (mouse insulinoma) cells are widely utilized [19, 20]. These β-cell lines provide a controlled system to evaluate the cytotoxic, oxidative, and metabolic effects of toxicants. Studies have demonstrated that exposure to Cd, As, Pb, and

Mn in INS-1 and MIN6 cells leads to decreased cell viability, reduced insulin secretion, altered gene expression, and increased oxidative stress. Such findings underscore the relevance of environmental toxicants in β-cell dysfunction and DM development [21].

This study aimed to investigate the cytotoxic and functional effects of four environmental heavy metals—Cd, As, Pb, and Mn—on pancreatic β-cell viability, oxidative stress, and insulin secretion using two *in vitro* models: MIN6 (mouse) and INS-1 (rat) β-cell lines. By comparing the responses of these two cell types to metal-induced toxicity, this study aimed to enhance the understanding of how environmental toxicants can contribute to β-cell dysfunction and the development of DM.

2. Materials and methods

2.1 Materials

Unless specified otherwise, all chemicals (including $CdCl_2$, $NaAsO_2$, $MnCl_2$, $PbCl_2$) and laboratory plastic wares were purchased from Sigma-Aldrich (Dorset, UK).

2.2 Cell culture

The mouse MIN6 cells, an insulin-secreting pancreatic β-cell line, were used in this study. The cells (<30 passages) were cultured in Dulbecco's Modified Eagle's Medium (DMEM) containing 15% heat-inactivated fetal bovine serum (FBS), 100 U/mL penicillin, and 0.1 mg/mL streptomycin. The cells were maintained at 37°C in a humidified incubator with 5% CO_2. MIN6 cells were split when 80–90% confluent, then were used for experiments.

INS-1 cells, a rat insulin-secreting pancreatic β-cell line, were cultured in RPMI 1640 medium, supplemented with 50 U/mL penicillin, 2 mM L-glutamine, 10% FBS, 1 mM sodium pyruvate, 50 μM β-mercaptoethanol, and 0.1 mg/mL streptomycin in a humidified atmosphere with 5% CO_2 at 37°C, based on the method of Asfari et al. [22]. INS-1 cells were split when 80–90% confluent, then were used for experiments.

2.3 Measurement of cell viability

MIN6 and INS-1 pancreatic β-cells were seeded in 96-well plates at a density of 2×10^4 cells per well and allowed to adhere under standard culture conditions. Once confluent, the cells were treated with varying concentrations of Cd, As, Pb, or Mn for 24 h. After exposure, the treatment medium was removed and replaced with fresh medium with 0.2 mg/mL of 3-(4,5-dimethylthiazol-2-yl)-2,5-diphenyl tetrazolium bromide (MTT). The cells were incubated for an additional 4 hours at 37°C to allow for the formation of formazan crystals by metabolically active cells. After incubation, the medium was carefully removed, and the resulting blue formazan crystals were solubilized by adding 100 μL of dimethyl sulfoxide (DMSO) to each well. Absorbance was measured at 570 nm using a microplate reader (BioTek μQuant Monochromatic Microplate Spectrophotometer, MTX Lab Systems, Inc., USA). Cell viability was shown as a percentage relative to the untreated control group.

2.4 Determination of intracellular reactive oxygen species (ROS)

Intracellular ROS levels in MIN6 and INS-1 pancreatic β-cells were measured using the cell-permeant probe 2′,7′-dichlorodihydrofluorescein diacetate (H_2DCFDA), according to the manufacturer's instructions. Briefly, cells from different treatment groups were harvested and washed three times with sterile phosphate-buffered saline (PBS) to remove residual culture media and extracellular contaminants. Following washing, the cells were incubated in the dark at 37°C for 90 minutes in PBS containing 10 μmol/L H_2DCFDA. After incubation, excess extracellular dye was removed by washing the cells three additional times with sterile PBS. The oxidation of H_2DCFDA to the fluorescent product 2′,7′-dichlorofluorescein (DCF) within the cells was used as an indicator of intracellular ROS production. Fluorescence intensity was measured using flow cytometry with excitation at 485 nm and emission detection at 525 nm. ROS levels were presented as relative fluorescence units, normalized to those of the control group treated with 0.01% DMSO. All measurements were performed in triplicate to ensure reproducibility.

2.5 Lipid peroxidation (MDA)

Lipid peroxidation in MIN6 and INS-1 pancreatic β-cells was measured by the detection of the endpoint product malondialdehyde (MDA), according to the manufacturer's instructions, using the MDA microplate assay kit from Cohesion Biosciences (London, UK). MDA levels in the cell culture supernatant were measured by colorimetric analysis at 532 and 600 nm. MDA concentrations were normalized to total protein content and expressed as nmol/mg protein.

2.6 Glucose-stimulated insulin secretion (GSIS)

MIN6 and INS-1 pancreatic β-cells were plated and maintained under standard culture conditions until they achieved suitable confluency for the GSIS assay. The cells were then washed twice with PBS and subsequently treated with Cd, As, Pb, or Mn for 24 h at specified concentrations. After treatment, the culture medium was discarded, and the cells were rinsed with PBS to remove any remaining metal ions. Next, the cells were incubated at 37°C in glucose- and serum-free DMEM, supplemented with 2 mM L-glutamine and 25 mM HEPES (pH 7.4), and adjusted to a final glucose concentration of 25 mM to stimulate insulin secretion. Following a 15-minute incubation, the supernatants containing secreted insulin were collected, and the cells were subsequently lysed using the method outlined by Cheng et al. [23]. Cell lysis was performed using an acid/ethanol solution (1.5:70 v/v%) to extract intracellular insulin for determining total insulin content. Both media samples and cell lysates were analyzed using a commercial insulin ELISA kit, and absorbance was measured at 450 nm using a microplate reader. Insulin secretion was normalized to the total insulin content of the cells to account for variations in cell number or viability. Each experimental condition was conducted in at least four biological replicates per metal concentration.

2.7 Statistical analysis

Data were expressed as means ± SEM. Statistical analysis was performed by GraphPad Prism 10.0 (GraphPad Software, San Diego, CA, USA) using one-way analysis of variance (ANOVA) and Tukey's multiple comparisons post hoc test to

DOI: http://dx.doi.org/10.5772/intechopen.1011942

compare the means of the experimental groups. Data represents duplicate measurements from three independent experiments. Groups that do not share the same letters are significantly different ($p < 0.05$).

3. Results

3.1 Cytotoxic effects of heavy metals on MIN6 and INS-1 pancreatic β cells

The impact of various heavy metals on the viability of MIN6 and INS-1 pancreatic β cells was assessed using the MTT assay. To evaluate whether these metals could synergistically enhance cytotoxicity, the cells were exposed to $CdCl_2$, $MnCl_2$, $NaAsO_2$, and $PbCl_2$ for 24 h at varying concentrations. A significant reduction in cell viability was observed at 2 μM concentrations of $CdCl_2$ and $NaAsO_2$, whereas $MnCl_2$ and $PbCl_2$ induced notable cytotoxicity at 5 μM in both cell lines (**Figures 1** and **2**).

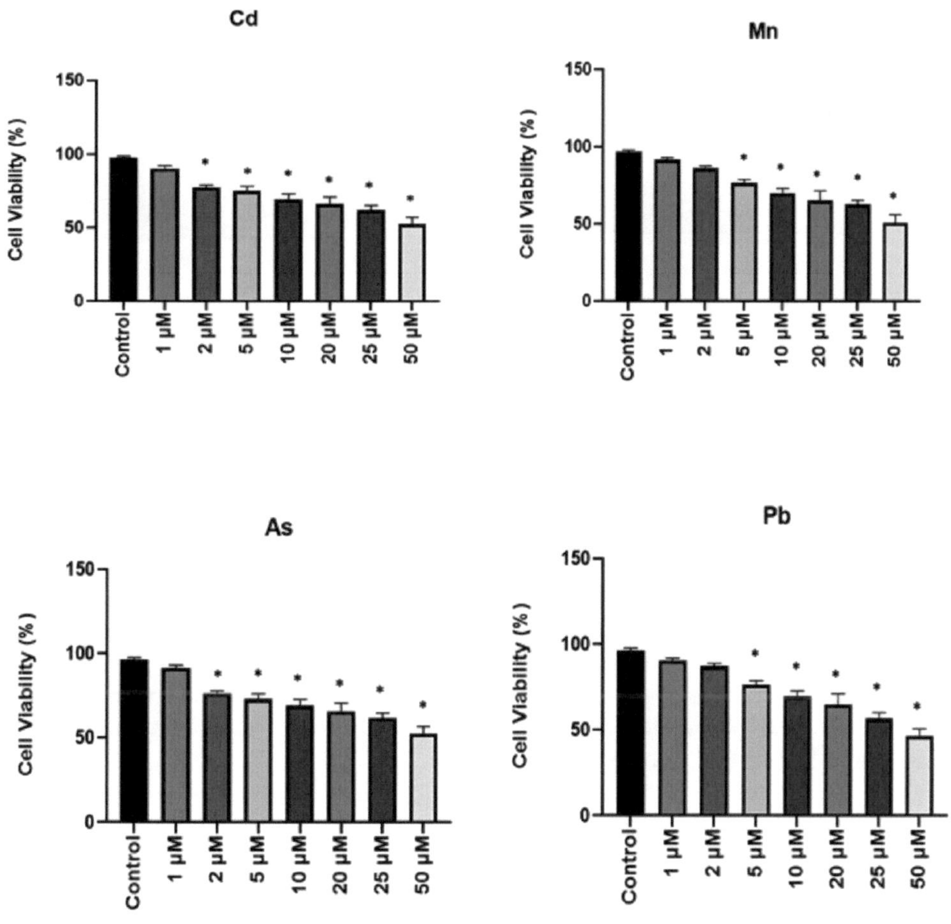

Figure 1.
Dose-dependent effect of heavy metals on MIN6 cell viability. Different doses of $CdCl_2$, $MnCl_2$, $NaAsO_2$, and $PbCl_2$ were exposed to MIN6 for 24 h. Data are presented as mean ± SEM, representing at least three independent experiments ($n = 3$). Statistical significance was determined using one-way ANOVA followed by Tukey's post hoc test, with $p < 0.05$ indicating significant differences between control and treatment groups.

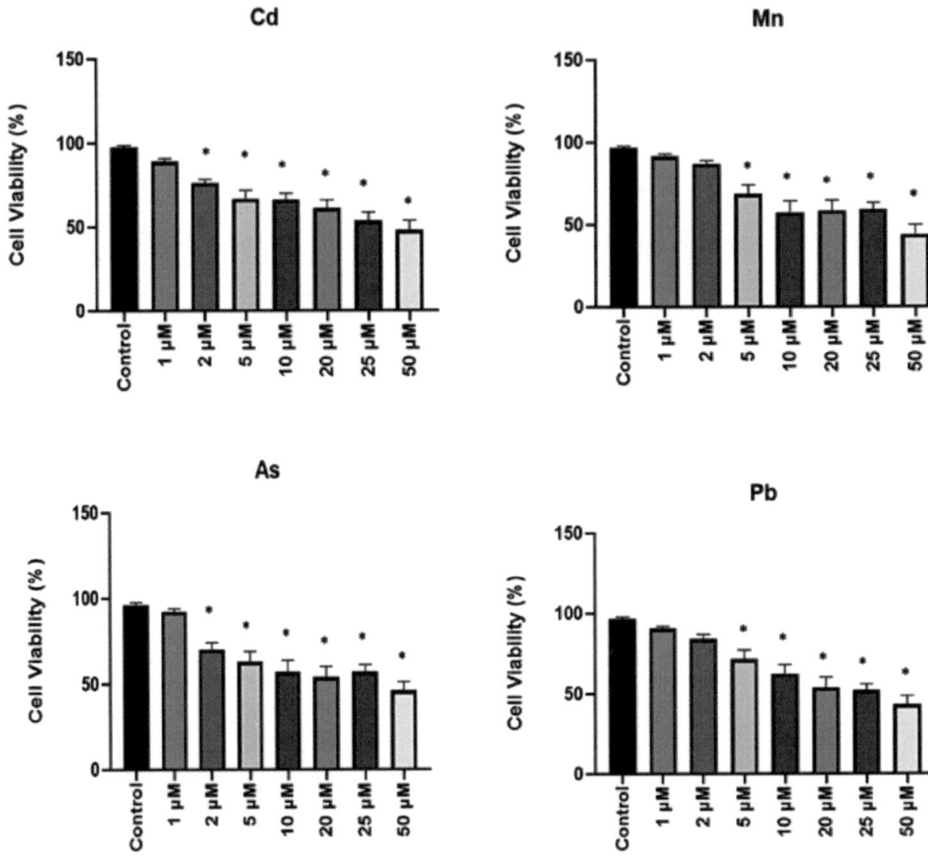

Figure 2.
Dose-dependent effect of heavy metals on INS-1 cell viability. Different doses of $CdCl_2$, $MnCl_2$, $NaAsO_2$, and $PbCl_2$ were exposed to MIN6 for 24 h. Data are presented as mean ± SEM, representing at least three independent experiments (n = 3). Statistical significance was determined using one-way ANOVA followed by Tukey's post hoc test, with $p < 0.05$ indicating significant differences between control and treatment groups.

3.2 Induction of oxidative stress by heavy metals

The influence of heavy metals on intracellular ROS levels and lipid peroxidation (MDA) was evaluated. As shown in **Figure 3A** and **B**, exposure to cytotoxic concentrations of the metals significantly elevated ROS levels in both cell lines compared to untreated controls. Lipid peroxidation, assessed by measuring malondialdehyde (MDA) levels, also increased markedly following treatment with 2 μM $CdCl_2$, 2 μM $NaAsO_2$, and 5 μM $MnCl_2$ or $PbCl_2$ (**Figure 3B**).

3.3 Effect of heavy metals on insulin secretion

To assess insulin secretion, MIN6 and INS-1 cells were incubated with 2.5 mM glucose (low glucose, negative control) or 16.7 mM glucose (high glucose, positive control). Cells treated with 2 μM $CdCl_2$, 2 μM $NaAsO_2$, 5 μM $MnCl_2$, or 5 μM $PbCl_2$ showed a significant decline in insulin release compared to the high glucose control (**Figure 4**), indicating a disruption in β-cell function.

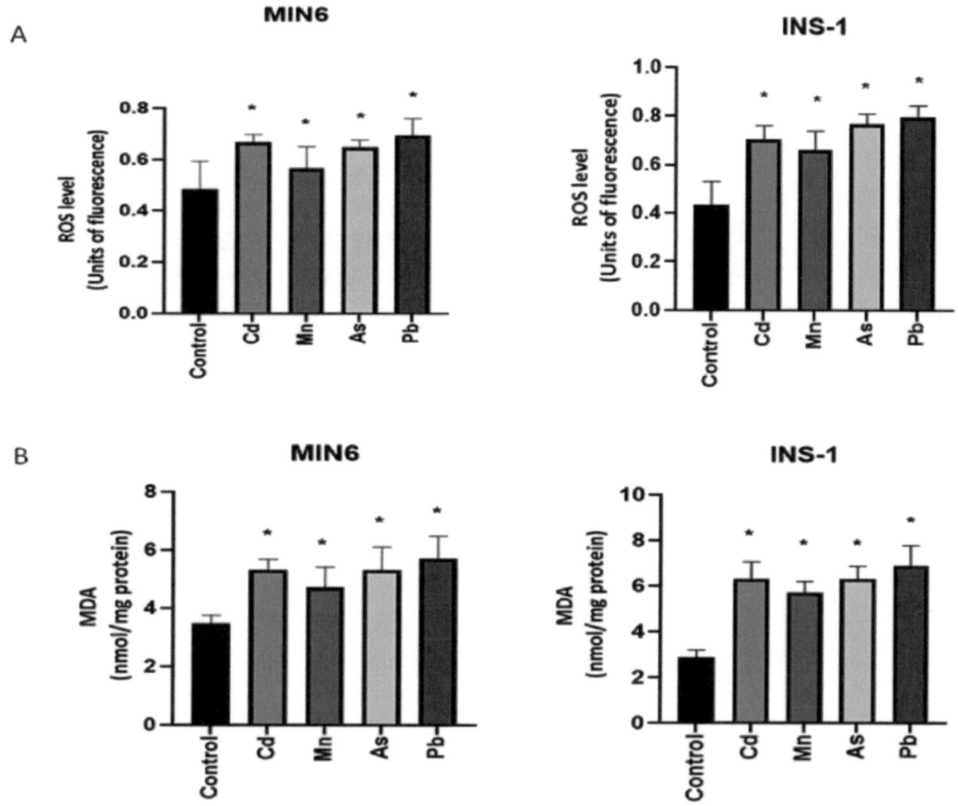

Figure 3.
Heavy metals increased intracellular ROS (A) and MDA (B) levels in MIN6 and INS-1 cells. The effect of heavy metals on intracellular levels of ROS (A) and (B) MDA in MIN6 and INS-1 cells was determined by assays. Data are presented as mean ± SEM, representing at least three independent experiments (n = 3). Statistical significance was determined using one-way ANOVA followed by Tukey's post hoc test, with p < 0.05 indicating significant differences between control and treatment groups.

4. Discussion

The present study investigated the cytotoxic effects of four environmentally relevant heavy metals: Cd, Mn, As, and Pb, on pancreatic β-cell function using two widely accepted *in vitro* models: MIN6 and INS-1 cells. Our findings demonstrate that exposure to these metals significantly impairs β-cell viability, disrupts GSIS, and elevates intracellular ROS, all of which are indicative of β-cell dysfunction and stress.

Cd was found to be the most toxic among the tested metals, consistent with previous reports highlighting its high affinity for sulfhydryl groups in proteins and its ability to disrupt cellular redox homeostasis [7]. *In vitro* studies using MIN6 and INS-1 cell lines have demonstrated that Cd reduces cell viability, disrupts insulin gene expression, and impairs insulin secretion through mechanisms involving mitochondrial dysfunction and the generation of reactive oxygen species [8, 24]. For example, Hong et al. [7] reported that Cd exposure at low micromolar concentrations significantly decreased insulin secretion in MIN6 cells by interfering with calcium homeostasis and mitochondrial potential.

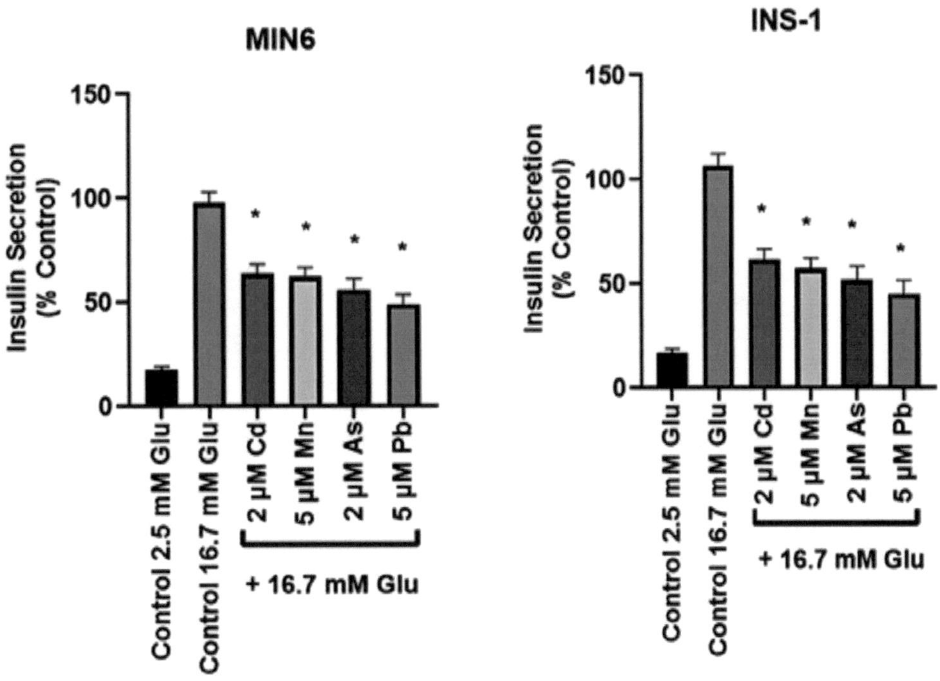

Figure 4.
The effect of heavy metals on insulin secretion in high glucose-treated MIN6 and INS-1 cells. Insulin secretion in MIN6 and INS-1 cells treated with high glucose (16.7 mM) was significantly reduced following exposure to heavy metals. Data are presented as mean ± SEM, representing at least three independent experiments (n = 3). Statistical significance was determined using one-way ANOVA followed by Tukey's post hoc test, with p < 0.05 indicating significant differences between control and treatment groups.

As, commonly present in contaminated drinking water, it has also been shown to damage β-cells. Chronic exposure to inorganic arsenic compounds such as $NaAsO_2$ has been linked to impaired insulin signaling and β-cell death. *In vitro*, exposure in MIN6 cells has been shown to reduce GSIS, increase oxidative stress markers, and alter β-cell gene expression, including key regulators such as Pdx1 and Ins1 [25]. Similarly, Sanchez-Soria et al. [26] demonstrated that arsenic trioxide induced mitochondrial fragmentation and suppressed insulin secretion in INS-1 cells, emphasizing the role of mitochondrial integrity in β-cell survival. Those results aligned with this study, supporting the hypothesis that chronic arsenic exposure contributes to insulin resistance and the development of DM.

Pb exposure led to moderate but significant reductions in both viability and insulin output. Pb is known to interfere with calcium signaling and disrupt mitochondrial activity, both of which are essential for insulin granule exocytosis. Furthermore, Pb-induced ROS production likely contributes to lipid peroxidation and membrane damage in β-cells. Our results align with previous studies, reporting an association between elevated blood lead levels and impaired glucose tolerance [11, 14].

Mn as an essential trace element, exerted cytotoxic effects at elevated concentrations. Mn-induced β-cell dysfunction is likely mediated through oxidative stress and mitochondrial dysregulation, consistent with earlier studies showing Mn overexposure impairs insulin signaling and alters antioxidant enzyme activities [15, 25]. Interestingly, the biphasic nature of Mn's biological activity—beneficial at physiological levels but harmful at toxic concentrations—highlights the need for precise regulation of metal exposure in maintaining β-cell integrity.

Comparative analysis of MIN6 and INS-1 cells revealed generally consistent responses across both models, though some variation in sensitivity was noted [27, 28]. This may reflect species-specific differences in metal uptake, detoxification pathways, or antioxidant capacity. Nonetheless, the use of both cell lines strengthens the translational relevance of our findings, suggesting that heavy metal exposure poses a substantial risk to β-cell function across mammalian systems [19, 27].

Overall, our study reinforces the emerging paradigm that environmental pollutants—particularly heavy metals—are important, but often overlooked, contributors to β-cell dysfunction and the pathogenesis of DM. The observed impairments in cell viability, insulin secretion, and redox balance underscore the need for stricter environmental controls and increased public health efforts to mitigate exposure to these toxic elements. Future research should aim to elucidate the precise molecular mechanisms underlying metal-induced β-cell damage and explore potential protective strategies, such as antioxidant supplementation or pharmacological intervention.

Acknowledgements

This chapter has been written by Tugba Kose.

Conflict of interest

The authors declare no conflict of interest.

Author details

Tugba Kose[1,2,3]

1 King's College London, London, UK

2 Hitit University, Çorum, Turkey

3 Quadram Institute Bioscience, Norwich, UK

*Address all correspondence to: tugba.kose@kcl.ac.uk

References

[1] Hectors TLM, Vanparys C, Van Der Ven K, Martens GA, Jorens PG, Van Gaal LF, et al. Environmental pollutants and type 2 diabetes: A review of mechanisms that can disrupt beta cell function. Diabetologia. 2011;**54**(6):1273-1290. DOI: 10.1007/s00125-011-2109-5

[2] Howard JL, Olszewska D. Pedogenesis, geochemical forms of heavy metals, and artifact weathering in an urban soil chronosequence, Detroit, Michigan. Environmental Pollution. 2011;**159**(3):754-761. DOI: 10.1016/j.envpol.2010.11.028

[3] Gastaldelli A, Gaggini M, DeFronzo RA. Role of adipose tissue insulin resistance in the natural history of type 2 diabetes: Results from the San Antonio metabolism study. Diabetes. 2017;**66**(4):815-822. DOI: 10.2337/db16-1167

[4] Edwards JR, Prozialeck WC. Cadmium, diabetes and chronic kidney disease. Toxicology and Applied Pharmacology. 2009;**238**(3):289-293. DOI: 1016/j.taap.2009.03.007

[5] Lei LJ, Jin TY, Zhou YF. Insulin expression in rats exposed to cadmium. Biomedical and Environmental Sciences. 2007;**20**(4):295-301. DOI: 2007/4/PDF/bes200704007

[6] Chen X, Zhu G, Gu S, Jin T, Shao C. Effects of cadmium on osteoblasts and osteoclasts in vitro. Environmental Toxicology and Pharmacology. 2009;**28**(2):232-236. DOI: 10.1016/j.etap.2009.04.010

[7] Hong H, He H, Lin X, Hayuehashi T, Xu J, Zhang J, et al. Cadmium exposure suppresses insulin secretion through mtROS-mediated mitochondrial dysfunction and inflammatory response in pancreatic beta cells. Journal of Trace Elements in Medicine and Biology. 2022;**71**:126952. DOI: 10.1016/j.jtemb.2022.126952

[8] Son HS, Kim SG, Suh BS, Park DU, Kim DS, Do YS, et al. Association of cadmium with diabetes in middle-aged residents of abandoned metal mines: The first health effect surveillance for residents in abandoned metal mines. Annals of Occupational and Environmental Medicine. 2015;**27**(1):4-11. DOI: 10.1186/s40557-015-0071-2

[9] Paul D, Kazy SK, Das BT, Gupta AK, Pal T, Sar P. Arsenic biotransformation and release by bacteria indigenous to arsenic contaminated groundwater. Bioresource Technology. 2015;**188**:14-23. DOI: 10.1016/j.biortech.2015.02.039

[10] Wang Y, Liu Y, Liu S, Wu B. Influence of iron on cytotoxicity and gene expression profiles induced by arsenic in HepG2 cells. International Journal of Environmental Research and Public Health. 2019;**16**(22):4484. DOI: 10.3390/ijerph16224484

[11] Yan LD, Rouzier V, Pierre JL, Lee MH, Muntner P, Parsons PJ, et al. High lead exposure associated with higher blood pressure in Haiti: A warning sign for low- income countries. Hypertension. 2022;**79**(1):283-290. DOI: 10.1161/hypertensionaha.121.1825

[12] Cricenti A. Different membrane modifications revealed by AFM/LFM after doping of pancreatic cells with Cd, Zn or Pb. Microsc Res Tech. 2003;**427**:422-427. DOI: 10.1063/1.1639729

[13] Girasole M, Cricenti A, Generosi R, Longo G, Pompeo G, Cotesta S, et al.

Different membrane modifications revealed by atomic force/lateral force microscopy after doping of human pancreatic cells with Cd, Zn, or Pb. Microscopy Research and Technique. 2007;**70**(10):912-917. DOI: 10.1002/jemt.20486

[14] Al Doghaither H, Elmorsy E, Al-Ghafari A, Ghulam J. Roles of oxidative stress, apoptosis, and inflammation in metal-induced dysfunction of beta pancreatic cells isolated from CD1 mice. Saudi Journal of Biological Sciences. 2021;**28**(1):651-663. DOI: 10.1016/j.sjbs.2020.10.056

[15] Peres TV, Schettinger MRC, Chen P, Carvalho F, Avila DS, Bowman AB, et al. Manganese-induced neurotoxicity: A review of its behavioral consequences and neuroprotective strategies. BMC Pharmacology and Toxicology. 2016;**17**(1). DOI: 10.1186/s40360-016-0099-0

[16] Li L, Yang X. The essential element manganese, oxidative stress, and metabolic diseases: Links and interactions. Oxidative Medicine and Cellular Longevity. 2018;**2018**(1):1-11. DOI: 10.1155/2018/7580707

[17] Dover EN, Patel NY, Stýblo M. Impact of in vitro heavy metal exposure on pancreatic β-cell function. Toxicology Letters. 2018;**299**:137-144. DOI: 10.1016/j.toxlet.2018.09.015

[18] Sun Z, Shao Y, Yan K, Yao T, Liu L, Sun F, et al. The link between trace metal elements and glucose metabolism: Evidence from zinc, copper, iron, and manganese-mediated metabolic regulation. Metabolites. 2023;**13**(10). DOI: 10.3390/metabo13101048

[19] Merglen A, Theander S, Rubi B, Chaffard G, Wollheim CB, Maechler P. Glucose sensitivity and metabolism-secretion coupling studied during two-year continuous culture in INS-1E Insulinoma cells. Endocrinology. 2004;**145**(2):667-678. DOI: 10.1210/en.2003-1099

[20] Luther MJ, Hauge-Evans A, Souza KLA, Jörns A, Lenzen S, Persaud SJ, et al. MIN6 β-cell interactions influence insulin secretory responses to nutrients and non-nutrients. Biochemical and Biophysical Research Communications. 2006;**343**(1):99-104. DOI: 10.1016/j.bbrc.2006.02.003

[21] Dinić S, Arambašić Jovanović J, Uskoković A, Mihailović M, Grdović N, Tolić A, et al. Oxidative stress-mediated beta cell death and dysfunction as a target for diabetes management. Frontiers in Endocrinology. 2022;**13**:1-20. DOI: 10.3389/fendo.2022.1006376

[22] Asfari M, De W, Nöel M, Holthuizen PE, Czernichow P. Insulin-like growth factor-II gene expression in a rat insulin-producing beta-cell line (INS-1) is regulated by glucose. Diabetologia. 1995;**38**(8):927-935. DOI: 10.1007/BF00400581

[23] Cheng KC, Li YX, Asakawa A, Ushikai M, Kato I, Sato Y, et al. Characterization of preptin-induced insulin secretion in pancreatic β-cells. Journal of Endocrinology. 2012;**215**(1):43-49. DOI: 10.1530/joe-12-0176

[24] Engström A, Michaëlsson K, Suwazono Y, Wolk A, Vahter M, Åkesson A. Long-term cadmium exposure and the association with bone mineral density and fractures in a population-based study among women. Journal of Bone and Mineral Research. 2011;**26**(3):486-495. DOI: 10.1002/jbmr.224

[25] Dover EN, Beck R, Huang MC, Douillet C, Wang Z, Klett EL, et al.

Arsenite and methylarsonite inhibit mitochondrial metabolism and glucose-stimulated insulin secretion in INS-1 832/13 β cells. Archives of Toxicology. 2018;**92**(2):693-704. DOI: 10.1007/s00204-017-2074-y

[26] Sanchez-Soria P, Broka D, Quach S, Hardwick RN, Cherrington NJ, Camenisch TD. Fetal exposure to arsenic results in hyperglycemia, hypercholesterolemia, and nonalcoholic fatty liver disease in adult mice. Journal of Toxicology and Health. 2014;**1**(1):1. DOI: 10.7243/2056-3779-1-1

[27] Chao X, Zhao F, Hu J, Yu Y, Xie R, Zhong J, et al. Comparative study of two common In vitro models for the pancreatic islet with MIN6. Tissue Engineering and Regenerative Medicine. 2023;**20**(1):127-141. DOI: 10.1007/s13770-022-00507-8

[28] Chen YW, Yang CY, Huang CF, Hung DZ, Leung YM, Liu SH. Heavy metals, islet function and diabetes development. Islets. 2009;**1**(3):169-176. DOI: 10.4161/isl.1.3.9262

Chapter 4

The Role of Emerging Environmental Contaminants on Alzheimer's Disease

İ. İpek Boşgelmez and Beyza Mertaş

Abstract

According to the latest data from WHO, about 57 million individuals worldwide were living with dementia in 2021, with 10 million new cases diagnosed each year. Alzheimer's disease (AD) accounts for approximately 60–80% of dementia cases and ranks as the seventh leading cause of death globally. Currently, the therapeutic options available for AD have limited effectiveness, and potential disease-modifying therapies are not widely adopted or reliably deemed safe. Therefore, implementing preventive strategies and raising public awareness about the relevant AD risk factors are crucial. Existing data delineate various risk factors for AD, encompassing non-modifiable factors such as age, genetic predisposition, and gender, alongside modifiable factors including environmental pollution and diet. This chapter aims to explore emerging environmental risk factors that contribute to AD, including air pollution, toxic elements, pesticides, microplastics, nanoplastics, endocrine disruptors, pharmaceuticals and personal care products, environmental disasters, and global climate change. The intricate and multifaceted nature of neurodegenerative disorders such as AD necessitates an interdisciplinary approach to unravel the underlying mechanisms. This involves the effective application of various omics techniques—such as genomics, transcriptomics, proteomics, metabolomics, and lipidomics—paired with advanced artificial intelligence (AI) methods, including machine learning and deep learning.

Keywords: Alzheimer's disease, environmental risk factors, air pollution, water pollution, soil pollution, microplastics and nanoplastics, toxic metals, pesticides, pharmaceuticals and personal care products, changes to the natural environment, environmental disasters, global climate change, endocrine disruptors, noise pollution, light pollution

1. Introduction

Alzheimer's disease (AD), first characterized by Dr. Alois Alzheimer in 1906, is a progressive neurodegenerative disorder marked by a progressive decline in cognitive functions and behavioral capabilities. It is recognized as the most common form of dementia and poses a growing challenge in the context of the aging global population. Currently, AD is an enduring and largely untreatable condition, with only a limited number of medications available, imposing a significant socio-economic burden [1, 2]. In 2021, AD and other dementias ranked as the seventh leading cause of mortality worldwide, accounting for approximately 1.8 million deaths. The mortality rate for AD is strongly correlated with aging (**Figure 1a**), particularly among individuals over 70 years of age [3]. Additionally, country-specific data highlight the global importance of this issue (**Figure 1b**). Furthermore, women are

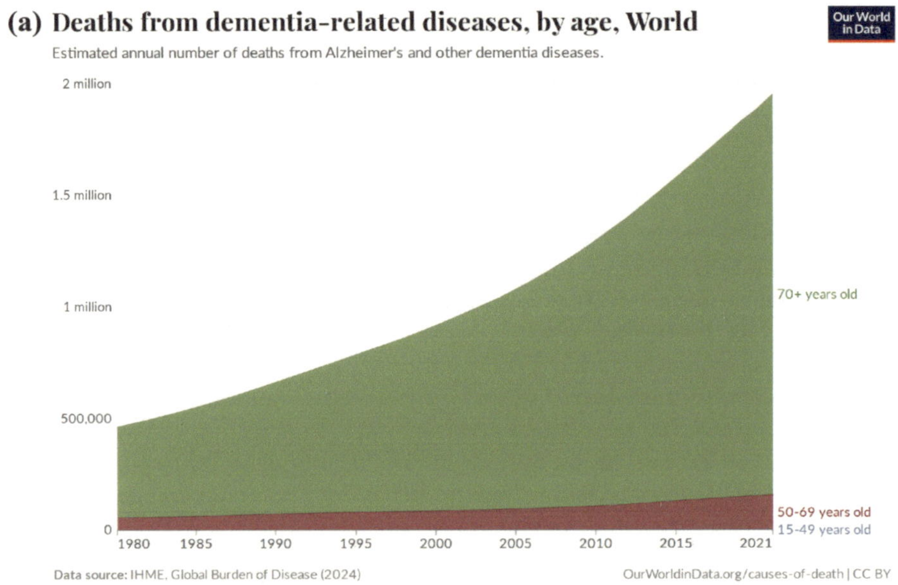

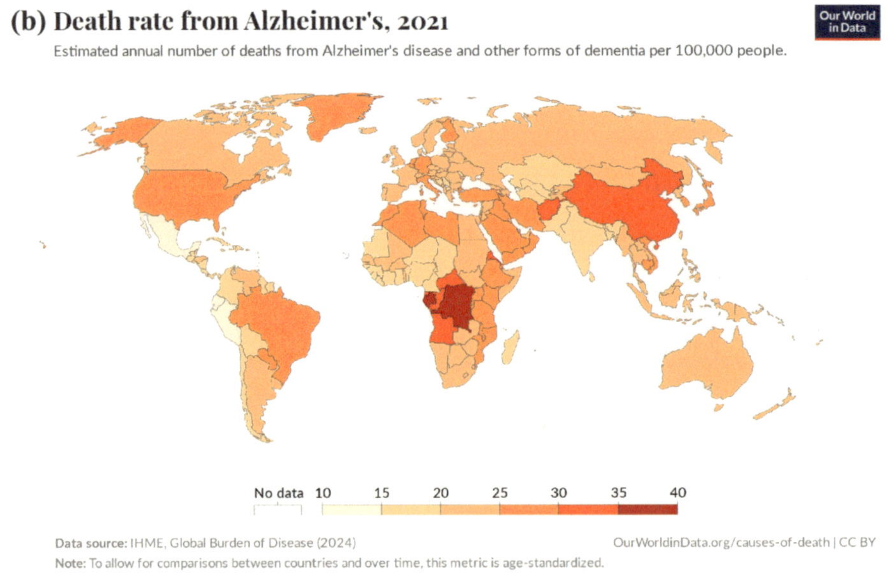

Figure 1.
(a) Mortality rate from AD and other dementias by age, (b) Global view of AD-related mortality across countries [3].

disproportionately impacted by dementia worldwide, comprising 68% of deaths related to AD and other dementias [4]. The hallmark features of AD include amyloid plaques—aggregates of amyloid-beta (Aβ) peptides—and neurofibrillary tangles, composed of hyperphosphorylated tau protein within the brain's neural structures. This pathological protein aggregation disrupts the functions and communication of neuronal networks, thereby accelerating the cognitive decline typically observed in disease progression.

2. An overview of risk factors and hypotheses

As illustrated in **Figure 2**, risk factors related to AD are categorized into two groups: "non-modifiable factors," such as genetics, gender, and aging; and "modifiable factors," including lifestyle, various diseases, and environmental pollution. The key point is that these modifiable factors can be targeted to potentially prevent or delay up to 45% of dementia cases. Currently, these factors are categorized according to the stages of life, as early life, midlife, and late life risk factors [5]. The constantly evolving landscape of related AD research results in the daily emergence of new risk factors and updates in clinical practice.

Various hypotheses related to AD (**Figure 3**), such as the amyloid, tau propagation, cholinergic, mitochondrial cascade, inflammatory, neurovascular, and metal ion hypotheses, have been proposed [6].

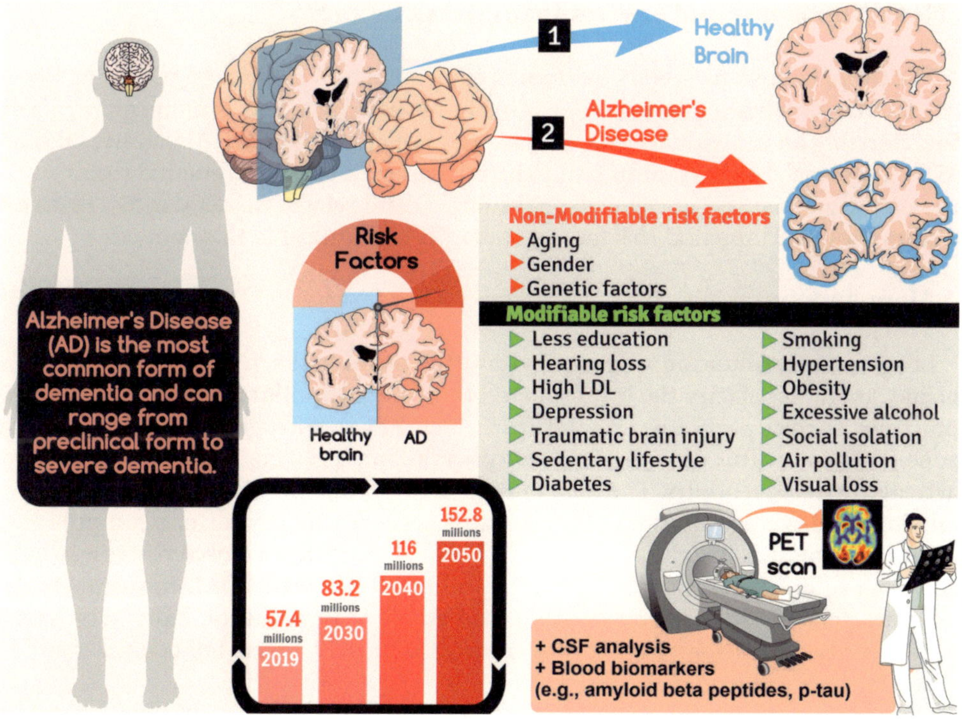

Figure 2.
Risk factors and other key points of AD.

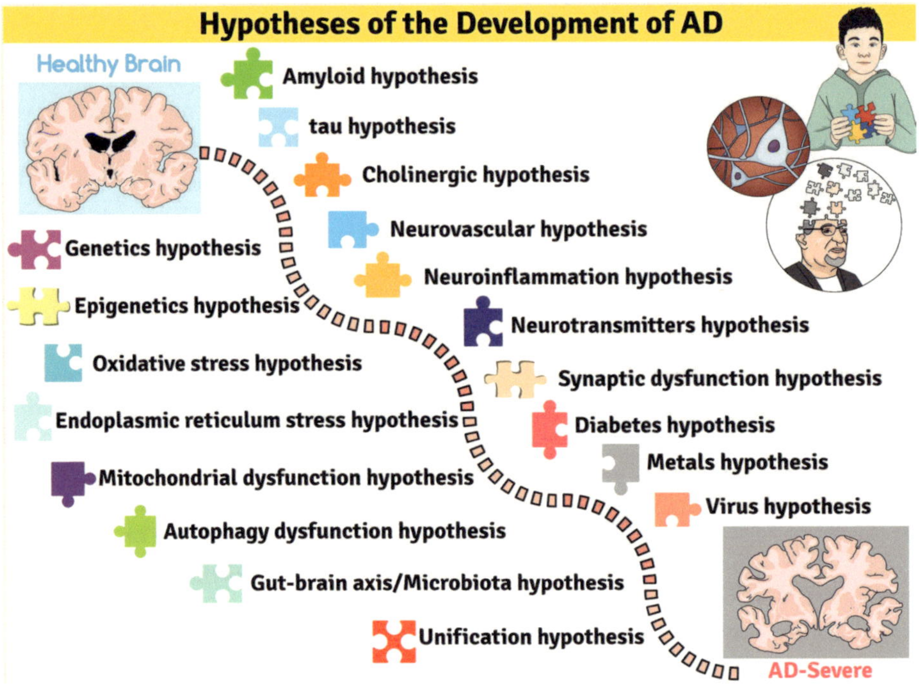

Figure 3.
Currently known hypotheses related to AD.

3. Neuroexposome and environmental risk factors

The term "exposome" refers to lifetime environmental exposures, including lifestyle factors, that begin prenatally [7]. Due to its variability and dynamism, precisely characterizing an individual's exposure history is challenging. An "Alzheimer's disease (AD) exposome" has been proposed to better understand environmental factors influencing genetic and non-genetic risks for AD and related dementias [8]. **Figure 4** outlines the environmental risk factors currently recognized in this context.

3.1 Air pollution

Long-term air pollution exposure is linked to health risks, including cognitive decline, as studies clarify the harmful effects of specific pollutants. Airborne contaminants, such as particulate matter ($PM_{2.5}$ and PM_{10}), nitrogen dioxide (NO_2), ozone (O_3), and sulfur dioxide (SO_2), may lead to impaired cognitive function, particularly in older adults. The data in **Figure 5a** [9] and **5b** [3] show air pollutant emissions and average annual $PM_{2.5}$ exposure, respectively, and offer a comprehensive overview of the global situation. Guo et al. reported a global rise in age-standardized mortality rates and disability-adjusted life years (DALYs) related to AD and other dementias, based on an analysis of ambient air pollution indicators—such as $PM_{2.5}$, NO_2, and O_3—and covariates from 1990 to 2019 across 149 countries and territories [10].

Over the past three decades, O_3 levels increased annually by 0.17%, while $PM_{2.5}$ and NO_2 decreased by 0.33% and 0.14%, respectively. A 10 μg/m^3 rise in $PM_{2.5}$ was associated with a 0.118 (95% CI: 0.060–0.175) increase in ASMR and a 0.966 (95%

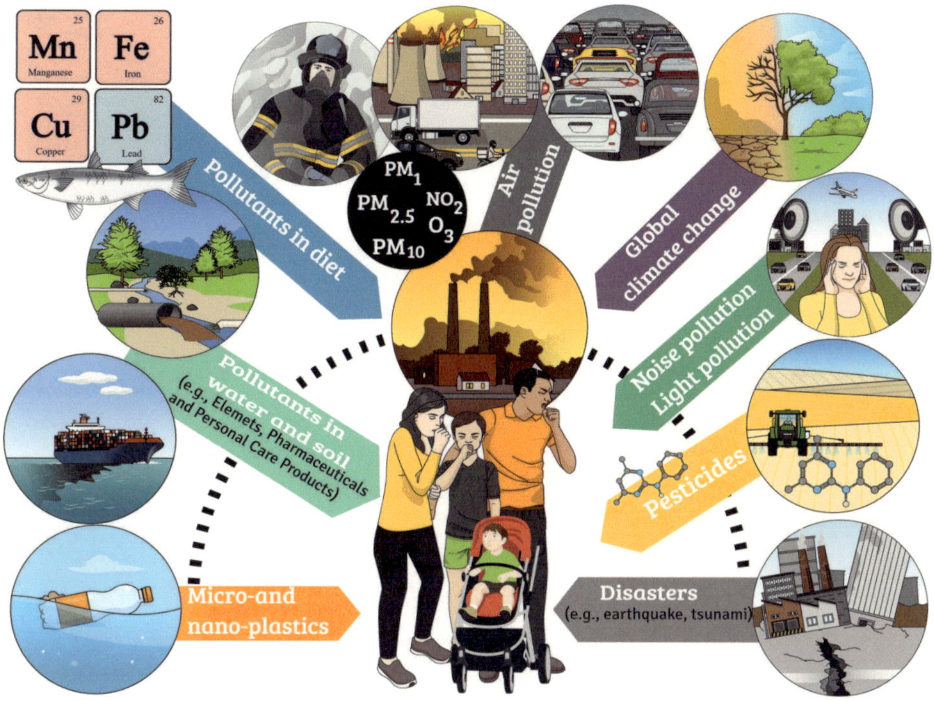

Figure 4.
A representation of proposed environmental risk factors on neurodegenerative diseases.

CI: 0.321–1.611) increase in DALYs. Similarly, every 10 μg/m^3 increase in O_3 correlated with a 0.112 rise in ASMR and a 1.068 rise in DALYs. Notably, stronger associations between O_3 and dementia were observed in the Global South compared to the Global North. Prolonged exposure to NO_2 has been linked to lower memory and executive function assessment scores. Specifically, a significant decline of −0.10 in memory performance has been observed for each interquartile range increase [11].

Increased particulate matter exposure is associated with higher risks of cognitive decline, supported by odds ratios (OR: 1.49 for $PM_{2.5}$; 1.30 for PM_{10}) [12]. A recent systematic review [13] across Europe, Asia, and North America links $PM_{2.5}$ and PM_{10} to behavioral issues in adults and the elderly, including olfactory dysfunction, cognitive deterioration, dementia, depression, and anxiety, with memory effects being most common. Some studies suggest gender-specific vulnerabilities, with women showing a higher incidence of adverse outcomes. Further research is needed to clarify the relationship between PM exposure and dementia risk.

Prolonged exposure to poor air quality is linked to neuroinflammation, immune response alterations, blood-brain barrier (BBB) disruption, and accumulation of Aβ-42 and α-synuclein, elevating risks of Alzheimer's and Parkinson's diseases, especially in *APOE e4* allele carriers. This early-life exposure potentially heightens the risk of developing neurodegenerative diseases later in life [14].

Formaldehyde has also been implicated in the pathogenesis of neurodegenerative diseases due to its mechanism of action, which is significantly associated with heightened accumulation of Aβ. Exposure to exogenous formaldehyde may exacerbate this process in individuals who demonstrate a predisposition to Aβ accumulation, influenced by factors such as age or genetic traits. The receptor for advanced glycation end

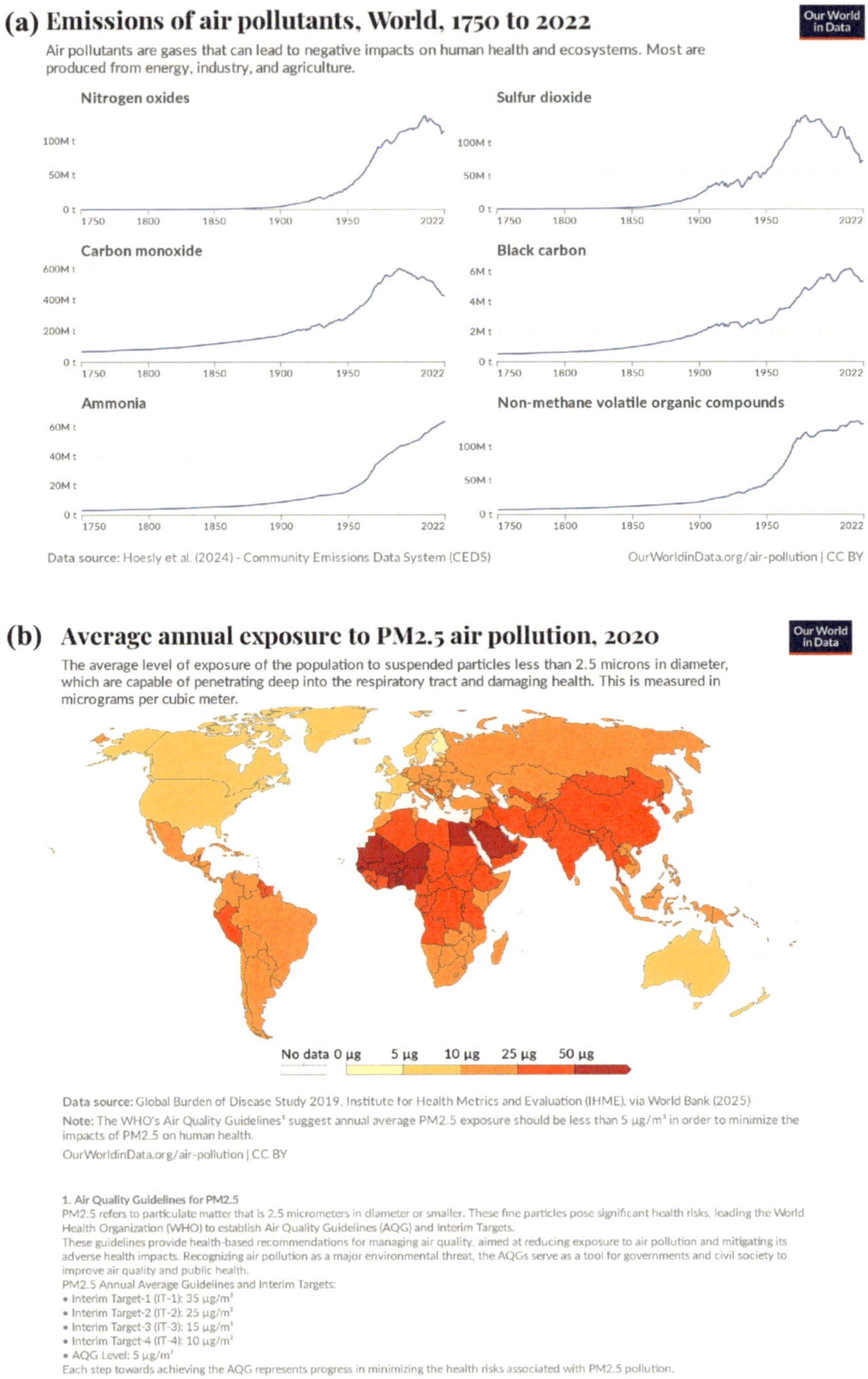

Figure 5.
(a) air pollutant emissions [9], (b) average annual exposure to $PM_{2.5}$ [3].

products (RAGE) is essential for the transport of Aβ across the BBB. The interaction of ligands with RAGE plays a crucial role in regulating the expression of the amyloid precursor protein (APP), a key component in the accumulation of Aβ. Endogenous formaldehyde accumulation within the body can result from impaired metabolic processes. In contrast, the accumulation of exogenous formaldehyde, which has been documented to surpass the maximum permissible concentration in various regions globally, may present more immediate and severe consequences [15]. Exposure to formaldehyde may lead to insulin deficiency, which impairs glucose metabolism and subsequently results in the accumulation of RAGE ligands, particularly advanced glycation end products (AGEs). The accumulation of glucose and the disruption of insulin-dependent biochemical signaling may trigger a cascade of reactions that promote neuroinflammation and various cellular disorders. Consequently, this increases the level of RAGE ligands in the system. The overexpression of RAGE at the BBB facilitates the transport of Aβ from the bloodstream into the brain. An increase in ligand-RAGE interactions subsequently upregulates the expression of the APP and beta-site amyloid precursor protein cleaving enzyme 1 (BACE1) genes, disrupting the equilibrium of APP processing and leading to the formation of elevated Aβ levels. The accumulation of Aβ contributes to the development of amyloid plaques. This phenomenon exhibits a cyclical nature; the deposition of amyloid plaques provokes neuroinflammation and diminishes neuroplasticity [15].

3.2 Water and soil pollution

Water pollution is a growing concern globally as the population and industrialization continue to rise. Contaminants detected in water sources include heavy metals such as lead (Pb), mercury (Hg), and arsenic (As), as well as pharmaceutical and cosmetic waste [16]. A study conducted in China found that an increase in water pollution resulted in worse mental health, with low-income participants being particularly vulnerable. Notably, the pollutants associated with adverse mental health outcomes were As, Hg, Pb, ammonia nitrogen (NH_3-N), volatile phenol, and chemical oxygen demand (COD). Researchers also reported that water treatment ameliorated mental health by 0.12 percent [17]. It is also worth noting that water is the primary source of exposure to inorganic As. In Project FRONTIER, the association between the current and long-term As exposure and neuropsychological functioning was examined. The study included 434 participants, with a mean long-term As exposure of 240.15 μg/L-years over 34 years. The approximate current As level in the area where participants reside was 6.33 μg/L. Researchers have reported that long-term, low-level exposure to As is associated with impairments in global cognition, immediate memory, language, processing speed, and executive functioning [18]. Another study hypothesized that psychoactive pharmaceuticals from drinking water can cross maternal biological barriers and induce neurological disorders, including AD, by changing gene and protein expression [19]. In their previous study, Kaushik et al. [20] treated human neuronal cells with valproate and a mixture of fluoxetine, venlafaxine, and carbamazepine, and they found almost a 2-fold change in expression of genes associated with AD such as nuclear protein 1 (*NUPR1*), dihydropyrimidinase related protein 2 (*DRP2*), and Thrombospondin-1 (*TSP1*). *NUPR1* is a gene that plays a role in cell apoptosis and regulation [21]. Both mixture and carbamazepine administration resulted in the upregulated expression of *NUPR1*, just as observed in AD patients [20]. Researchers suggest *NUPR1* is related to brain damage [22], while Xu et al. found inhibition of *NUPR1* improves learning and memory *in vivo* and reduces apoptosis [23]. Another downregulated gene in both AD and, due to the mixture and carbamazepine administration, is *DRP2* [20, 24]. A current study found that *DRP2* may be involved in regulating neuronal dedifferentiation during memory formation in complex conditioned tasks. This process appears to increase the pool of neuronal precursor cells, which can then differentiate in a targeted manner to encode newly acquired behaviors [25].

TSP-1 gene expression is downregulated in AD patients and *in vivo* models. One study indicates that Aβ reduces astrocytic *TSP-1* secretion [26], while another suggests this gene offers protection against Aβ-induced mitochondrial fission, dysfunction, and apoptosis [27]. Taken together, these results indicate that mixtures of pharmaceutical waste in drinking water pose a significant risk factor for AD through multiple mechanisms. However, there are limited studies that investigate the association between pharmaceutical waste and AD. More demographic studies are crucial for taking effective measures and analyzing levels of heavy metals, especially As, as well as cosmetic and pharmaceutical waste, in drinking water.

The Food and Agriculture Organization of the United Nations (FAO) defines soil pollution as "the presence in the soil of a chemical or substance out of place and/or present at a higher than normal concentration that has adverse effects on any non-targeted organism" [28]. According to the FAO, several sources contribute to soil pollution, including pesticides, plastic and healthcare waste, naturally occurring asbestos, organic contaminants, transportation, and trace elements [29]. Li et al. found that soil As concentration was significantly associated with AD mortality rates, whereas no such association was observed for Pb, Cd, and Hg. The researchers noted the lack of investigation into As levels in drinking water as a limitation and emphasized the necessity of incorporating water exposure assessments in future studies on As and AD prevalence, given the potential for metal exchange between soil and water [30]. An analysis of data from all 48 US states examined the correlation between AD mortality rates and 41 trace elements. Results showed that soil selenium levels had the strongest inverse relationship with AD mortality rates, while soil tin concentrations were most notably linked to a decrease in AD mortality growth, followed by sulfur. The study also posited that selenium and sulfur levels in soil could account for approximately 20.8% of the observed spatial variation in AD mortality across these states [31]. Overall, these results suggest that soil composition can be both a risk and a protective factor. Studies examining specific trace elements and their association with AD could help determine beneficial components and improve soil quality. Furthermore, increasing public awareness and promoting effective agricultural practices can serve as a long-term and effective intervention.

3.3 Noise and light pollution

Alongside air pollution, noise pollution—such as traffic noise and around-the-clock noise at work—has become a significant public health concern. Noise pollution is an emerging health threat globally, affecting approximately 132 million people in Europe. According to the European Environment Agency, more than 30% of Europeans are exposed to noise levels known to increase the risk of cardiovascular, metabolic, and mental health diseases [32]. Noise can increase the risk of both auditory and non-auditory health conditions, including cardiovascular diseases, diabetes, and cognitive/neurodegenerative disorders [33, 34]. Specific occupational and routine environments may expose individuals to prolonged noise, potentially leading to emotional and cognitive problems linked to neurobiological changes resembling those seen in AD. Growing research in epidemiology and experimental studies underscores the connection between ongoing noise exposure and declining cognitive function.

When exposed to noise, the hypothalamic-pituitary-adrenal axis and the sympathetic nervous system are activated, resulting in the secretion of stress hormones, including catecholamines and cortisol. Chronic noise exposure precipitates sustained inflammation and oxidative damage, which may contribute to various health issues. This underscores the importance of mitigating noise pollution to protect public health. Furthermore, the roles of inflammation and oxidative stress in noise-induced vascular dysfunction, circadian rhythm disturbances, accelerated aging, neuroinflammation, and alterations in the microbiome are significant, emphasizing their interconnected nature [35].

In a rat model of chronic noise-induced cognitive impairment [36], the pathological condition of the hippocampus and levels of ferroptosis were examined using Western blotting and immunohistochemical techniques. Subsequent bioinformatics analysis identified several key genes, including the *retinoic acid receptor responder-2* gene, which has been proposed as a protective factor in AD. This gene, acting upstream of ferroptosis, was suggested as a potential target for preventing and treating noise-induced cognitive impairment. In another study examining the molecular mechanisms behind cognitive impairment induced by continuous noise exposure, researchers found decreased expression of the *serum/glucocorticoid-regulated kinase 1 (SGK1)* gene and its associated protein. This dysregulation inhibited the intracellular *PI3K/SGK1/Foxo3* pathway, resulting in increased expression of apoptotic proteins, including B-cell lymphoma-2 (Bcl-2), Bcl-2-associated X protein (*Bax*), Fas Ligand (*FasL*), and tumor necrosis factor (*TNF*)-related apoptosis-inducing ligand (*TRAIL*) [37]. However, considering the intricate interplay of various risk factors, further data are essential to clarify the causal relationship between noise pollution and neurodegenerative diseases [38].

3.4 Examples of known and emerging toxicants

3.4.1 Endocrine disruptors

According to WHO [39], "An endocrine disruptor is an exogenous substance or mixture that alters function(s) of the endocrine system and consequently causes adverse health effects in an intact organism, its progeny, or (sub)populations." Whether synthetic or natural in origin, their action involves mimicking or blocking the actions of endogenous hormones. A meta-analysis of studies involving 286,610 participants identified endocrine-disrupting chemicals (EDCs) as significant risk factors for neurodegenerative diseases, with high exposure to EDC mixtures associated with a 1.03-fold increased risk of AD. A positive correlation between AD risk and polychlorinated biphenyls (PCBs) was also reported [40]. A study found that prenatal BPA exposure alters gene expression in offspring's hippocampus, affecting 1633 genes in males and 2780 in females compared to controls. These genes are involved in inflammation, synaptic transmission, neuritogenesis, and neurodevelopment, and are associated with AD and related neurological disorders such as cognitive impairment and tauopathies. BPA exposure also increased nuclear factor-κB (NF-κB) levels exclusively in males, indicating sex-specific pathways. It also differentially affected BACE1 expression—upregulating it in males with no change in females—suggesting sex-dependent effects on amyloid processing [41].

Taken together, these findings underscore the need to consider sex differences and prenatal exposure when investigating the association between AD and EDCs. Exposure to EDCs begins prenatally and continues throughout life; thus, their cumulative effects on AD must be considered and investigated. Therefore, more epidemiological and *in vivo* studies are crucial not only to improve regulatory policies regarding these pollutants but also to make effective interventions to raise public awareness.

3.4.2 Pesticides

The rise in the global population and the growing need for food and pest management have resulted in extensive pesticide use, raising awareness of the potential link between pesticides and AD. In particular, the association between prolonged exposure to low doses of pesticides and AD, as well as other neurodegenerative disorders, has garnered significant attention. A meta-analysis of seven studies reported an OR of 1.34 (95% CI: 1.08–1.67), supporting the hypothesis that pesticides could be a risk factor for AD [42]. A significant positive correlation between pesticide exposure and AD was observed in high-use regions in Spain, with an OR of 2.09 compared to lower-exposure areas. Female subjects exhibited a higher risk (OR: 2.27), suggesting gender-specific susceptibility to pesticide neurotoxicity. These findings highlight the importance of incorporating gender considerations in research and public health policies targeting environmental neurodegenerative risks [43]. Hayden et al. [44] reported that after adjusting for baseline age, gender, education, *APOE* ε4 status, and baseline Modified Mini-Mental State Examination scores (MMSE), Cox proportional hazards (CPH) models indicated increased risks among pesticide-exposed individuals for all-cause dementia (HR 1.38, 95% CI 1.09–1.76) and for AD (HR 1.42, 95% CI 1.06–1.91). The risk of AD associated with exposure to organophosphates (hazard ratio [HR] 1.53, 95% confidence interval [CI] 1.05–2.23) was slightly higher than that linked to organochlorines (HR 1.49, 95% CI 0.99–2.24), which was nearly statistically significant. In a CPH study of 26 agricultural activities, increased AD risk correlated with high pesticide use. The hazard ratios were higher in crop farming, fruit arboriculture, and viticulture [3.72 (95% CI: 3.47–3.98), 1.36 (1.15–1.62), and 1.29 (1.18–1.42), respectively], while lower risks were observed among breeders [45].

Despite bans over 50 years ago due to environmental persistence, the pesticide dichlorodiphenyltrichloroethane (DDT) and its metabolite, dichlorodiphenyldichloroethylene (DDE), are still detectable in some countries, pointing to ongoing concerns. Both compounds elevate APP levels in human neuroblastoma cells, reinforcing a mechanistic connection. Elevated serum DDE is significantly associated with a 3.8-fold increased risk of AD, with a correlation coefficient of 0.95 between serum and brain DDE levels. Specifically, within the subgroup exposed to the highest tertile of DDE, carriers of the *APOE* ε4 allele scored approximately 1.75 points lower on the MMSE compared to those with the *APOE* ε3 allele. In this context, detecting individuals with high levels of DDE and carrying an APOE ε4 allele may enable early identification of some AD cases [46]. Further mechanistic investigations revealed that exposure to DDT significantly upregulated APP mRNA and protein levels in SH-SY5Y cells, primary neuronal cultures, and both wild-type (C57BL/6J) and 3xTG-AD mouse models. An increase in secreted Aβ levels was also detected in SH-SY5Y cells, with this effect being counteracted by the sodium channel blocker tetrodotoxin. Transgenic flies and 3xTG-AD mice exhibited heightened Aβ pathology following DDT exposure, indicating a possible link between DDT and Aβ-aggregation. Moreover, levels of synaptic markers such as synaptophysin and PSD95 were decreased in the cortices of 3xTG-AD mice [47].

Bartholomew et al. [48] reported that administration of glyphosate to 3xTg-AD mice resulted in decreased survival rates, increased thigmotaxis in the Morris water maze, and significant elevations in the enzyme BACE1, which is involved in amyloidogenic processing. Additionally, there was an increase in insoluble Aβ-42 fractions, greater plaque load and enlarged plaques, as well as elevated levels of pTau at epitopes Threonine 181, Serine 396, and the AT8 epitope (Serine 202, Threonine 205). Pro- and anti-inflammatory cytokines and chemokines increased and persisted in the brain tissue of both 3xTg-AD and non-Tg groups, as well as in the peripheral blood plasma of 3xTg-AD. Additionally, the primary metabolite of glyphosate, aminomethylphosphonic acid, was detected in the brains of 3xTg-AD and non-Tg mice exposed to glyphosate, even after a 6-month recovery period.

Recent *in vitro* research [49] suggests that pyrimethanil, a fungicide, accelerates Aβ42 aggregation by promoting the formation of small oligomers during the lag phase and inducing β-sheet-structured aggregates. In the presence of preformed seeds, pyrimethanil has a dual role, fragmenting fibrils and promoting aggregation, likely through interactions with smaller seeds. Pyrimethanil shows a higher affinity for fibrils than for monomers, thereby weakening the interactions between monomers and fibrils.

3.4.3 Toxic metals and other elements

Various elements such as aluminum (Al), arsenic (As), iron (Fe), manganese (Mn), lead (Pb), copper (Cu), and cadmium (Cd) have garnered academic interest in this context [50–53]. Some of these metals have been proposed to interfere with key neural processes, including oxidative stress regulation, mitochondrial function, and autophagy, promoting neurodegeneration. Specifically, it has been posited that As influences tau phosphorylation and Aβ accumulation; Mn affects glutamate regulation and excitotoxicity; and Pb and Cd impair mitochondrial bioenergetics and induce cellular senescence, elucidating their roles in AD pathogenesis [52].

3.4.4 Microplastics and nanoplastics

Given the extensive utilization of plastics across various sectors—including food and beverage packaging, pharmaceuticals, dietary supplements, infant feeding bottles, and medical devices—exposure to plastic materials in everyday life has become nearly unavoidable. Considering that human exposure to plastics begins prenatally, it is essential to examine the degree of bioaccumulation within the human body, as well as its distribution patterns and the overall fate. A recent post-mortem study found that brain concentrations of micro- and nanoplastics (MNPs) are 7–30 times greater than in the liver and kidney. Furthermore, brain samples from decedents in 2024 showed approximately 50% higher concentrations of MNPs compared to those from 2016. Markedly increased levels of MNPs were detected in the brain tissues of individuals diagnosed with dementia, with further accumulation observed in cerebrovascular walls and immune cells. Researchers have emphasized that a comprehensive understanding of the pathways of exposure, absorption, and elimination of MNPs, as well as their potential harmful effects—especially on the brain—is essential [54].

A recent study investigated the effects of prenatal nano-plastic exposure and found that nano-polystyrene-exposed rats' offspring exhibited upregulation of pregnancy-zone protein (PZP), fibronectin 1 (FN1), and alpha-2-macroglobulin (α-2 M) in the hippocampus. Researchers suggested that these changes suggest potential neural damage in the experimental group. They also found downregulation of kinesin family member 21A (KIF21A), stathmin (STMN2), dematin actin-binding protein

(DMTN), and MAGUK scaffold protein discs large (DLG1) in the nano-polystyrene-exposed rats' offspring. They hypothesized that the downregulation of DMTN increased the risk of brain tumors, while the downregulation of STMN2 and KIF21A was associated with impaired synaptic development in offspring. Additionally, they observed downregulation of DLG1, which plays a key role in neuronal development and synaptic regulation in offspring. Given this, the results suggest prenatal exposure to nanoplastics (NPs) represents a neurodevelopmental risk factor through several proteins linked to neural and synaptic development and functions [55]. Another study administered an environmentally relevant dose (10 mg/kg/day) of NPs to APP/PS1 mice for 28 days and reported that NPs significantly elevated the number and varying sizes of Aβ plaques. Additionally, they found that NPs impair cellular responses by decreasing the number and activation of microglia and astrocytes and suggested that NPs exposure might exacerbate AD progression.

Researchers hypothesize that microglia are the primary cells mediating dose-dependent NP uptake in the AD brain, providing insight into AD pathology [56]. Concurrently, co-exposure to ozone and polystyrene induces anxiety-like behaviors, cognitive deficits, and neuronal and BBB damage. This exposure elevates neuro-inflammation, evidenced by increased pro-inflammatory cytokines (TNF-α, IL-6, and IL-1β) and reduced anti-inflammatory factors (TGF-β, YM-1, and IL-10). It also enhances pyroptosis markers (caspase-1, GSDMD-N, IL-18, and IL-1β) and exacerbates oxidative stress, indicated by decreased superoxide dismutase (SOD) and increased 4-hydroxynonenal. Notably, exposure to either pollutant alone yielded minimal effects. These findings suggest synergistic interactions between NPs and air pollutants in promoting AD onset and progression [57].

Bashirova et al. examined the impact of nanoparticle size (50 and 140 nm) and concentration (0, 10, 50, and 100 ppm) of polyethylene terephthalate (PET) on Aβ1-40 fibrillation. The findings indicate that PET50nm accelerates fibrillation more than PET140nm across all concentrations. Fibrillation time increases with concentration but levels off at higher amounts. PET NPs at 50 nm and 100 ppm promote Aβ aggregation by enhancing fibril growth and nucleation [58].

3.4.5 Pharmaceuticals and personal care products

Pharmaceutical products and their metabolites, specifically non-steroidal anti-inflammatory drugs (NSAIDs), beta-blockers, hormones, antidepressants, and antiepileptics, are frequently detected in the environment [59]. These substances may be regarded as emerging risk factors for AD. According to the WHO, one of the main limitations when assessing the hazardous effects of waste pharmaceuticals is that very few studies and monitoring programs are available [60]. Moreover, pharmaceutical waste profiles differ internationally in both quantity and quality. Further research is required to evaluate how changes in pharmaceutical waste composition affect public health and to pinpoint at-risk groups. Nonetheless, it is reasonable to assume that as the population ages and pollution rises, pharmaceutical use and waste are expected to increase. Monitoring pharmaceutical waste, implementing preventive strategies, and enhancing public awareness are critical measures to mitigate its potential hazards effectively.

Personal care products constitute an emerging environmental risk factor, accumulating gradually over time. The most prevalent among these are fragrances, UV filters in sunscreens, chemicals in hair dyes, preservatives, insect repellents, and bactericidal/disinfectant agents [61]. Studies have documented the ubiquitous presence of pharmaceuticals and personal care products (PPCPs) across various water resources, including surface water, groundwater, wastewater, drinking water, and oceans; a typical example is triclosan [62]. The widespread production and consumption of PPCPs have led to an increase in their release into the environment. If adequate measures are not taken to control their environmental release, their potential adverse effects on public health are likely to become more pronounced over time. These adverse effects might be attributed to their specific mechanisms of action or to certain excipients included in the formulation.

A recent study [63] investigated the association between cognitive function and exposure to phenols, parabens, and phthalates widely used in cosmetic ingredients. In total, nine compounds across various categories were included in the analysis: BPA and triclosan (TCS) as phenolics; methylparaben (MPB) and ethylparaben (EPB) as parabens; and mono-2-ethyl-5-carboxypentyl phthalate (MECP), mono-ethyl phthalate (MEOH), mono-2-ethylhexyl phthalate (MEHP), mono-isobutyl phthalate (MiBP), and mono-benzyl phthalate (MBzP) as phthalates. The findings indicate a significant correlation with cognitive impairment for each of the nine exposures. Researchers emphasized that the cognitive function of the male population is more affected by the compounds examined in the study. Among all the compounds, MECP exposure was found to have the most significant influence [63]. An AD model in *Caenorhabditis elegans* revealed that early-life and prolonged exposure to di(2-ethylhexyl) phthalate (DEHP), the second most frequently identified phthalate in cosmetic products, increases intracellular reactive oxygen species (ROS) levels and Aβ deposition [64, 65]. DEHP has been shown to upregulate bec-1, which is associated with apoptosis and autophagy and causes apoptotic cell death when activated [64, 66]. They also hypothesized that upregulation of bec-1 leads to increased accumulation of lysosome-related organelles (LROs) through Aβ-induced autophagosome formation, emphasizing the significance of the autophagy–lysosomal degradation pathway in response to DEHP exposure [64].

In addition to phthalates, exposure to heavy metals *via* personal care products may constitute a significant risk factor for AD. Notably, aluminum—an element extensively found in cosmetics, including eye shadows, mascaras, lipsticks, and antiperspirants—raises particular concern due to its pervasive presence [67]. Even though several studies have shown a relationship between aluminum exposure and AD, there is insufficient evidence to conclusively establish a link between aluminum exposure from personal care products and the development or progression of the disease [68, 69]. In the study by Rusina et al. [70], the mean aluminum concentration in the brains of AD patients was approximately four times higher than that of healthy controls. A post-mortem study with familial AD patients detected co-localization of aluminum and neurofibrillary tangles in their frontal cortex, temporal, and parietal lobes [68]. Another study investigated aluminum-regulated mechanisms, resulting in abnormal tau phosphorylation, and hypothesized that aluminum can modulate tau hyperphosphorylation *via* protein kinases and phosphatases that take part in the phosphorylation and production of the tau protein, such as glycogen synthase kinase 3 beta (GSK-3β) and PP2A. They also found that aluminum influences ubiquitin-proteasome pathway (UPP), which modulates tau hyperphosphorylation by selectively recognizing and degrading misfolded and aggregated tau proteins. In that study, aluminum doses specifically correlated with phosphorylated tau proteins such as pThr181, pThr231, and pSer396 [69]. Furthermore, a study shows that aluminum is cytotoxic and promotes oxidative stress, with Aβ42 significantly amplifying these effects, nearly doubling ROS-positive cells. These findings suggest aluminum's role in AD, likely through oxidative stress and cytotoxicity, and highlight its synergistic interaction with Aβ [71]. Taken together, the literature suggests that aluminum may be a risk factor for AD, acting through multiple mechanisms, influencing tau hyperphosphorylation *via* GSK-3β, UPP, and protein phosphatase 2A (PP2A), as well as inducing oxidative stress and cell death alongside Aβ42 [69, 71]. Although some excipients used in PPCPs are associated with causing disease onset and exacerbating prognosis, it remains unclear whether the concentrations in these products are sufficient to exert such effects, emphasizing the need for further studies in this area.

3.5 Changes to the natural environment

3.5.1 Global climate change

Recent studies revealed a potential link between climate change and the increased incidence of neurodegenerative diseases, including AD [72, 73]. Wei et al. [73] found that a 1.5°C increase in the summer mean temperature was associated with a 12% increase in dementia-related hospital admissions [72]. In line with these findings, Culqui et al. (2017) reported that when the maximum daily temperature surpassed the 34°C heatwave threshold, emergency hospital admissions for AD increased by 23.1%, with this association observed exclusively for temperatures exceeding this threshold [74]. A recent study emphasizes the growing threat of extreme heat to older adults living with AD and related dementias. The study indicates that higher temperatures significantly increase hospital admissions for AD and related dementias, with researchers urging clinicians and policymakers to address the risks of extreme heat for individuals with dementia and raise public awareness [75]. Another study found a marked increase in mortality due to AD and other forms of dementia during and after heatwave events. Researchers have underscored the urgent need for targeted public health interventions for AD and other dementia patients, noting that the implementation of appropriate heatwave response policies could significantly reduce heat-related mortality [76]. A study conducted in the United Kingdom estimated that each 1°C increase in high temperature is associated with a 4.5% rise in dementia-related hospital admissions. Also in the study, researchers considered two potential future emissions scenarios: a low emissions scenario, in which global greenhouse gas (GHG) emissions are significantly reduced under a firm global mitigation policy, and a high emissions scenario, where GHG emissions continue to rise with minimal mitigation efforts, alongside increasing wealth and population. In the high emissions scenario, they predicted a 194% increase in 2030 and a 294% increase in 2040, corresponding to approximately 360 admissions in 2030 and 482 admissions in 2040, compared to 122 admissions in 2009. In the low emissions scenario, heat-attributable hospital admissions were predicted to rise by 214% in 2030 and 263% in 2040. In absolute numbers, this equates to approximately 357 heat-related admissions in 2030 and 412 admissions in 2040, compared to 114 in 2009 [77]. Although several studies suggest a link between climate change and AD, the mechanisms behind this association remain unclear. One potential mechanistic pathway through which climate change may influence the onset or progression of AD is mediated by age-related physiological changes that impair thermoregulatory efficiency. As a result of decreased basal metabolic rate, reduced muscle mass, and altered vasoconstrictor responses, older adults exhibit increased sensitivity to temperature variations and a diminished capacity for thermoregulatory adaptation [78, 79]. Another potential mechanism concerns the substantial anatomical overlap between specific brain regions involved in altered thermal perception and social cognition. This anatomical convergence suggests that thermoregulatory homeostasis may be impaired in mental diseases, which could help explain the increased sensitivity of individuals with dementia to climate change [80].

3.5.2 Environmental disasters and related loss

Environmental disasters are multidimensional risk factors for AD as they include psychological and physical trauma, heightened stress, loss of relatives and friends, financial loss, and migration. A meta-analysis reported that natural disasters significantly increase the risk of AD, all-cause dementia, and cognitive decline. Researchers emphasized that hurricanes, heat waves, and earthquakes with tsunamis are associated with a heightened risk of dementia and cognitive decline compared to other natural disasters, and they attributed this increased risk to their varying combinations of physical, psychological, and social factors [81].

A study investigated dementia risk after the 2011 Great East Japan Earthquake and tsunami and found that the loss of housing is significantly associated with a three-year decline in cognitive performance, and disasters exacerbate dementia symptoms. Researchers highlighted that depression onset and deteriorated social relationships might be potential mechanisms linking cognitive decline with the loss of housing. Interestingly, there was no significant association reported between dementia and the loss of relatives or friends [82]. However, another study conducted in Utah found that participants who faced three or more deaths of family members during adulthood, which might occur due to natural disasters, had double the risk of developing AD [83]. Every element and combination of the aftermath of disasters represents a risk factor whose significance might vary individually. When studying the link between AD and natural disasters, it is crucial to recognize these consequences as key risk factors and create supportive environments for affected individuals. The findings highlight the importance of exploring how environmental disasters influence diseases across various cultures and regions. More global research is needed to better understand the geographic, regional, and cultural factors involved.

Considering AD within the framework of natural disasters is essential, as both patients and caregivers encounter distinct challenges in these circumstances. A study reported that 96.3% of caregivers of AD and related dementia patients expressed a need for additional information on emergency planning. During disaster evacuations, caregivers reported challenges related to stigma and privacy, which may exacerbate patients' behavioral symptoms [84]. Given this, raising public awareness and organizing educational training programs for emergencies and disasters could benefit patients, families, and caregivers alike. Additionally, environmental hazards, such as unanticipated pollutant exposures, further complicate such scenarios.

4. Conclusion and future perspectives

In view of the complex nature of neurodegenerative diseases, including AD, a growing list of disciplines in addition to neurology, epidemiology, public health, and gerontology have started to contribute to the field. It is widely accepted that investigating novel biomarkers and drug targets is crucial for advancing the prevention and treatment of AD. While the APOE ε4 allele is a primary genetic risk factor for AD, recent research indicates its association with Parkinson's disease, frontotemporal dementia, and amyotrophic lateral sclerosis. Additionally, a five-protein panel—SPC25, NEFL, S100A13, TBCA, and LRRN1—has been identified as a predictor of APOE ε4 status independently of clinical diagnoses [85]. Therefore, in addition to the aforementioned disciplines, a number of related fields, including, but not limited to, toxicology, pharmacology, and ecology, should take part in well-designed, controlled studies to shed light in the sources of exposure, specific mechanisms as well as inter-relationship between the potential mechanisms, exposure models and other required points that remain to be fully elucidated. In this context, realizing AI's promise in AD research requires concerted efforts across diverse sectors and fields. Harnessing AI's full potential in AD research—such as developing non-invasive digital biomarkers, exposure monitoring *via* wearable sensors, early detection, patient stratification, and enhanced clinical trial efficiency—necessitates multidisciplinary collaboration [86].

Conflict of interest

The authors declare no conflict of interest.

Notes/thanks/other declarations

The authors express their gratitude to all researchers involved in AD studies, along with the patients and their families, for their essential contributions in investigating risk factors and exploring new treatments. The authors apologize to colleagues whose work cannot be cited due to space constraints.

Author details

İ. İpek Boşgelmez[1]* and Beyza Mertaş[2]

1 Faculty of Pharmacy, Department of Toxicology, Erciyes University, Kayseri, Türkiye

2 Faculty of Pharmacy, Department of Pharmacology, Düzce University, Düzce, Türkiye

*Address all correspondence to: ipekbosgelmez@gmail.com; ibosgelmez@erciyes.edu.tr

References

[1] Alzheimer's Association Report. Alzheimer's disease facts and figures. Alzheimer's & Dementia: The Journal of the Alzheimer's Association. 2025;**21**:e70235. DOI: 10.1002/alz.70235

[2] World Health Organization. WHO & World Health Organization: WHO. Geneva, Switzerland: Dementia; 2025. Available from: https://www.who.int/news-room/fact-sheets/detail/dementia

[3] IHME, Global Burden of Disease (2024) – With minor processing by our world in data. Death rate from Alzheimer's. In: Global Burden of Disease - Deaths and DALYs. Oxford, UK: IHME, Global Burden of Disease; 2025. Available from: https://archive.ourworldindata.org/20250624-125417/grapher/dementia-death-rates.html [Accessed: June 24, 2025]

[4] World Health Organization. WHO & World Health Organization: WHO. The Top 10 Causes of Death. Geneva, Switzerland: WHO; 2024. Available from: https://www.who.int/news-room/fact-sheets/detail/the-top-10-causes-of-death

[5] Livingston G, Huntley J, Liu KY, Costafreda SG, Selbæk G, Alladi S, et al. Dementia prevention, intervention, and care: 2024 report of the lancet standing commission. Lancet. 2024;**404**:572-628. DOI: 10.1016/S0140-6736(24)01296-0

[6] Liu PP, Xie Y, Meng XY, Kang JS. History and progress of hypotheses and clinical trials for Alzheimer's disease. Signal Transduction and Targeted Therapy. 2019;**4**:29. DOI: 10.1038/s41392-019-0063-8. Erratum in: Signal Transduct Target Ther. 2019;4:37. doi: 10.1038/s41392-019-0071-8

[7] Wild CP. Complementing the genome with an "exposome": The outstanding challenge of environmental exposure measurement in molecular epidemiology. Cancer Epidemiology, Biomarkers & Prevention. 2005;**14**(8):1847-1850. DOI: 10.1158/1055-9965.EPI-05-0456

[8] Finch CE, Kulminski AM. The Alzheimer's disease Exposome. Alzheimer's & Dementia. 2019;**15**(9):1123-1132. DOI: 10.1016/j.jalz.2019.06.3914

[9] Hoesly R, Smith SJ, Prime N, Ahsan H, Suchyta H, O'Rourke P, et al. Community Emissions Data System (CEDS) v_2024_07_08. Release Emission Data [Original Data Set]. DOI: 10.5281/zenodo.12803197. Retrieved from: Our World in Data. Available from: https://archive.ourworldindata.org/20250909-093708/grapher/so-emissions-by-world-region-in-million-tonnes.html [Accessed: September 9, 2025]

[10] Guo C, Wu D, Yang J, Lu X, Chen XY, Ma J, et al. Ambient air pollution and Alzheimer's disease and other dementias: A global study between 1990 and 2019. BMC Public Health. 2025;**25**(1):371. DOI: 10.1186/s12889-025-21600-2

[11] Wood D, Evangelopoulos D, Beevers S, Kitwiroon N, Demakakos P, Katsouyanni K. Exposure to ambient air pollution and cognitive function: An analysis of the English longitudinal study of ageing cohort. Environmental Health. 2024;**23**(1):35. DOI: 10.1186/s12940-024-01075-1

[12] Meo SA, Shaikh N, Alotaibi M, AlWabel AA, Alqumaidi H. Effect of air pollutants particulate matter (PM2.5, PM10), sulfur dioxide (SO2) and ozone

(O3) on cognitive health. Scientific Reports. 2024;**14**(1):19616. DOI: 10.1038/s41598-024-70646-6

[13] Cativiela-Campos B, Ruiz-Sobremazas D, Rodulfo-Cárdenas R, Barrasa A, Sánchez-Santed F, Colomina MT, et al. What are the consequences of PM air pollution exposure on elderly behavior? A systematic review. Environmental Pollution. 2025;**375**:126279. DOI: 10.1016/j.envpol.2025.126279

[14] Calderón-Garcidueñas L, Solt AC, Henríquez-Roldán C, et al. Long-term air pollution exposure is associated with neuroinflammation, an altered innate immune response, blood-brain barrier disruption, ultrafine particulate deposition, and accumulation of amyloid beta-42 and alpha-synuclein in children and young adults. Toxicologic Pathology. 2008;**36**(2):289-310. DOI: 10.1177/0192623307313011

[15] Mikhailov IG, Mikhailova MS, Shuvaev AN, Gorina YV, Belozor OS. RAGE-mediated effects of formaldehyde in Alzheimer's disease. Biochemistry (Mosc). 2025;**90**(3):334-348. DOI: 10.1134/S0006297924604593

[16] Tota M, Karska J, Kowalski S, Piątek N, Pszczołowska M, Mazur K, et al. Environmental pollution and extreme weather conditions: Insights into the effect on mental health. Frontiers in Psychiatry. 2024;**15**:1389051. DOI: 10.3389/fpsyt.2024.1389051

[17] Wang Q, Yang Z. Industrial water pollution, water environment treatment, and health risks in China. Environmental Pollution. 2016;**218**:358-365. DOI: 10.1016/j.envpol.2016.07.011

[18] O'Bryant SE, Edwards M, Menon CV, Gong G, Barber R. Long-term low-level arsenic exposure is associated with poorer neuropsychological functioning: A project FRONTIER study. International Journal of Environmental Research and Public Health. 2011;**8**(3):861-874. DOI: 10.3390/ijerph8030861

[19] Kaushik G, Thomas MA. The potential association of psychoactive pharmaceuticals in the environment with human neurological disorders. Sustainable Chemistry and Pharmacy. 2019;**13**:100148. DOI: 10.1016/j.scp.2019.100148

[20] Kaushik G, Xia Y, Yang L, Thomas MA. Psychoactive pharmaceuticals at environmental concentrations induce in vitro gene expression associated with neurological disorders. BMC Genomics. 2016;**17**(Suppl. 3):435. DOI: 10.1186/s12864-016-2784-1

[21] Chowdhury UR, Samant RS, Fodstad O, Shevde LA. Emerging role of nuclear protein 1 (NUPR1) in cancer biology. Cancer Metastasis Reviews. 2009;**28**(1-2):225-232. DOI: 10.1007/s10555-009-9183-x

[22] Cui Y, Yang G, Li H, Sun J, Liu X, Xia X. Reduced expression of NUPR1 alleviates epilepsy progression via attenuating ER stress. Biochemical and Biophysical Research Communications. 2024;**730**:150365. DOI: 10.1016/j.bbrc.2024.150365

[23] Xu L, Xu Q, Xu F, Zhang W, Chen Q, Wu H, et al. MicroRNA-325-3p prevents sevoflurane-induced learning and memory impairment by inhibiting Nupr1 and C/EBPβ/IGFBP5 signaling in rats. Aging (Albany NY). 2020;**12**(6):5209-5220. DOI: 10.18632/aging.102942

[24] Lubec G, Nonaka M, Krapfenbauer K, Gratzer M, Cairns N, Fountoulakis M. Expression of the dihydropyrimidinase related protein 2 (DRP-2) in down syndrome and Alzheimer's disease

brain is downregulated at the mRNA and dysregulated at the protein level. Journal of Neural Transmission. Supplementum. 1999;**57**:161-177. DOI: 10.1007/978-3-7091-6380-1_10

[25] Mekhtiev AA, Asadova SM. Impact of dihydropyrimidinase-related protein 2 in memory formation on rats and its possible role in neuronal back remodeling. IBRO Neuroscience Reports. 2024;**16**:155-161. DOI: 10.1016/j.ibneur.2024.01.001

[26] Son SM, Nam DW, Cha MY, Kim KH, Byun J, Ryu H, et al. Thrombospondin-1 prevents amyloid beta-mediated synaptic pathology in Alzheimer's disease. Neurobiology of Aging. 2015;**36**(12):3214-3227. DOI: 10.1016/j.neurobiolaging.2015.09.005

[27] Kang S, Byun J, Son SM, Mook-Jung I. Thrombospondin-1 protects against aβ-induced mitochondrial fragmentation and dysfunction in hippocampal cells. Cell Death Discovery. 2018;**4**:31. DOI: 10.1038/s41420-017-0023-4

[28] Rodríguez-Eugenio N, McLaughlin M, Pennock D. Soil Pollution: A Hidden Reality. Rome: Food and Agriculture Organization of the United Nations; 2018

[29] FAO, UNEP. Global Assessment of Soil Pollution: Report [Internet]. Rome: Food and Agriculture Organization of the United Nations; 2021. DOI: 10.4060/cb4894en [Accessed: July 16, 2025]

[30] Li XL, Zhan RQ, Zheng W, Jiang H, Zhang DF, Shen XL. Positive association between soil arsenic concentration and mortality from Alzheimer's disease in mainland China. Journal of Trace Elements in Medicine and Biology. 2020;**59**:126452. DOI: 10.1016/j.jtemb.2020.126452

[31] Sun H. Associations of spatial disparities of Alzheimer's disease mortality rates with soil selenium and sulfur concentrations and four common risk factors in the United States. Journal of Alzheimer's Disease. 2017;**58**(3):897-907. DOI: 10.3233/JAD-170059

[32] European Environment Agency. Environmental Noise in Europe 2025: Summary for Policymakers. Luxembourg: Publications Office of the European Union; 2025. DOI: 10.2800/2287869

[33] Basner M, Babisch W, Davis A, Brink M, Clark C, Janssen S, et al. Auditory and non-auditory effects of noise on health. Lancet. 2014;**383**(9925):1325-1332. DOI: 10.1016/S0140-6736(13)61613-X

[34] Münzel T, Sørensen M, Daiber A. Transportation noise pollution and cardiovascular disease. Nature Reviews. Cardiology. 2021;**18**(9):619-636. DOI: 10.1038/s41569-021-00532-5

[35] Arregi A, Vegas O, Lertxundi A, Silva A, Ferreira I, Bereziartua A, et al. Road traffic noise exposure and its impact on health: Evidence from animal and human studies-chronic stress, inflammation, and oxidative stress as key components of the complex downstream pathway underlying noise-induced non-auditory health effects. Environmental Science and Pollution Research International. 2024;**31**(34):46820-46839. DOI: 10.1007/s11356-024-33973-9

[36] Ma J, Zhang J, Ou Z, Ren Y, Wu K, Zhang Y, et al. Chronic noise exposure induces Alzheimer's disease-like neuropathology and cognitive impairment via ferroptosis in rat hippocampus. Environmental Health and Preventive Medicine. 2024;**29**:50. DOI: 10.1265/ehpm.24-00126

[37] Fu Y, Zheng P, She X, Zhu Y, Fu B, Ma K, et al. Around-the-clock noise exposure induces hippocampus apoptosis and subsequent cognitive impairment via the PI3K/SGK1/Foxo3 signaling pathway. Journal of Translational Medicine. 2025;**23**(1):613. DOI: 10.1186/s12967-025-06501-7

[38] Kuntić M, Hahad O, Münzel T, Daiber A. Crosstalk between oxidative stress and inflammation caused by noise and air pollution-implications for neurodegenerative diseases. Antioxidants (Basel). 2024;**13**(3):266. DOI: 10.3390/antiox13030266

[39] International Programme on Chemical Safety. Global Assessment on the State of the Science of Endocrine Disruptors. Geneva, Switzerland: World Health Organization; 2002. Available from: https://iris.who.int/handle/10665/67357

[40] Wang C, Xu J, Pan K, Xu Y, Yu J. Relationship between endocrine disruptors and neurodegenerative diseases: Systematic review and meta-analysis. iScience. 2025;**28**(7):112779. DOI: 10.1016/j.isci.2025.112779

[41] Sukjamnong S, Thongkorn S, Kanlayaprasit S, Saeliw T, Hussem K, Warayanon W, et al. Prenatal exposure to bisphenol a alters the transcriptome-interactome profiles of genes associated with Alzheimer's disease in the offspring hippocampus. Scientific Reports. 2020;**10**(1):9487. DOI: 10.1038/s41598-020-65229-0

[42] Yan D, Zhang Y, Liu L, Yan H. Pesticide exposure and risk of Alzheimer's disease: A systematic review and meta-analysis. Scientific Reports. 2016;**6**:32222. DOI: 10.1038/srep32222

[43] Ruiz-González C, Román P, Rueda-Ruzafa L, Cardona D, Requena M, Alarcón R. Environmental pesticide exposure and Alzheimer's disease in southern Spain: A cross-sectional study. Psychiatry Research. 2024;**337**:115932. DOI: 10.1016/j.psychres.2024.115932

[44] Hayden KM, Norton MC, Darcey D, Ostbye T, Zandi PP, Breitner JC, et al. Cache County study investigators. Occupational exposure to pesticides increases the risk of incident AD: The Cache County study. Neurology. 2010;**74**(19):1524-1530. DOI: 10.1212/WNL.0b013e3181dd4423

[45] Petit P, Gondard E, Gandon G, Moreaud O, Sauvée M, Bonneterre V. Agricultural activities and risk of Alzheimer's disease: The TRACTOR project, a nationwide retrospective cohort study. European Journal of Epidemiology. 2024;**39**(3):271-287. DOI: 10.1007/s10654-023-01079-0. Erratum in: Eur J Epidemiol. 2024;39(5):569. doi: 10.1007/s10654-024-01116-6

[46] Richardson JR, Roy A, Shalat SL, von Stein RT, Hossain MM, Buckley B, et al. Elevated serum pesticide levels and risk for Alzheimer disease. JAMA Neurology. 2014;**71**(3):284-290. DOI: 10.1001/jamaneurol.2013.6030

[47] Eid A, Mhatre-Winters I, Sammoura FM, Edler MK, von Stein R, Hossain MM, et al. Effects of DDT on amyloid precursor protein levels and amyloid Beta pathology: Mechanistic links to Alzheimer's disease risk. Environmental Health Perspectives. 2022;**130**(8):87005. DOI: 10.1289/EHP10576

[48] Bartholomew SK, Winslow W, Sharma R, Pathak KV, Tallino S, Judd JM, et al. Glyphosate exposure exacerbates neuroinflammation and Alzheimer's disease-like pathology despite a 6-month recovery period in mice. Journal of

Neuroinflammation. 2024;**21**(1):316. DOI: 10.1186/s12974-024-03290-6

[49] Meyer N, Arroyo N, Roustan L, Janot JM, Perrier V, Torrent J, et al. Effect of pyrimethanil on aβ42 aggregation mechanisms revealed at single entity level and molecular dynamic simulations. Biophysical Chemistry. 2025;**325**:107471. DOI: 10.1016/j.bpc.2025.107471

[50] Campbell A. The potential role of aluminium in Alzheimer's disease. Nephrology, Dialysis, Transplantation. 2002;**17**(Suppl. 2):17-20. DOI: 10.1093/ndt/17.suppl_2.17

[51] Dhapola R, Sharma P, Kumari S, Bhatti JS, HariKrishnaReddy D. Environmental toxins and Alzheimer's disease: A comprehensive analysis of pathogenic mechanisms and therapeutic modulation. Molecular Neurobiology. 2024;**61**(6):3657-3677. DOI: 10.1007/s12035-023-03805-x

[52] Ahmed G, Rahaman MS, Perez E, Khan KM. Associations of environmental exposure to arsenic, manganese, Lead, and cadmium with Alzheimer's disease: A review of recent evidence from mechanistic studies. Journal of Xenobiotics. 2025;**15**(2):47. DOI: 10.3390/jox15020047

[53] Rashid F, Khan KM, Saiprakash S, Ahmed G, Sultana R, Parvez F, et al. Epidemiological evidence on the associations of metal exposure with Alzheimer's disease and related dementias among elderly women. Journal of Clinical Medicine. 2025;**14**(11):3776. DOI: 10.3390/jcm14113776

[54] Nihart AJ, Garcia MA, El Hayek E, Liu R, Olewine M, Kingston JD, et al. Bioaccumulation of microplastics in decedent human brains. Nature Medicine. 2025;**31**(4):1114-1119. DOI: 10.1038/s41591-024-03453-1. Erratum in: Nat Med. 2025;31(4):1367. doi: 10.1038/s41591-025-03675-x

[55] Chen J, Zhang Y, Liu X, Li K, Liu H, Lai W, et al. Effects of exposure to nano-plastic drinking during pregnancy on cognitive related proteins in offspring of SD rats. Environmental Pollutants and Bioavailability. 2023;**36**(1):2292104. DOI: 10.1080/26395940.2023.2292104

[56] Yu H, Zhao Z, Li H, Han Y, Li H, Cui C, et al. Nanoplastics exposure exacerbates aβ plaque deposition in Alzheimer's disease mice by inducing microglia pyroptosis. Ecotoxicology and Environmental Safety. 2025;**299**:118379. DOI: 10.1016/j.ecoenv.2025.118379

[57] Dai A, Liu X, Chen Y, Wang Y, Qi H, Zeng Y, et al. Co-exposure to ozone and polystyrene nanoplastic exacerbates cognitive impairment and anxiety-like behavior by regulating neuronal pyroptosis in mice. Environment International. 2025;**199**:109501. DOI: 10.1016/j.envint.2025.109501

[58] Bashirova N, Schölzel F, Hornig D, Scheidt HA, Krueger M, Salvan G, et al. The effect of polyethylene terephthalate nanoplastics on amyloid-β peptide fibrillation. Molecules. 2025;**30**(7):1432. DOI: 10.3390/molecules30071432

[59] Ribeiro AR, Castro PML, Tiritan ME. Environmental fate of chiral pharmaceuticals: Determination, degradation and toxicity. In: Lichtfouse E, Schwarzbauer J, Robert D, editors. Environmental Chemistry for a Sustainable World. Dordrecht, Netherlands: Springer; 2012. pp. 3-45. DOI: 10.1007/978-94-007-2439-6_1

[60] World Health Organization. Pharmaceuticals in Drinking-Water: Situation Report. Geneva: World Health Organization; 2012. 52 p. ISBN: 9789241502085. Available from:

https://www.who.int/publications/i/item/9789241502085

[61] Daughton CG, Ternes TA. Pharmaceuticals and personal care products in the environment: Agents of subtle change? Environmental Health Perspectives. 1999;**107**(Suppl. 6):907-938. DOI: 10.1289/ehp.99107s6907

[62] Ricart M, Guasch H, Alberch M, Barceló D, Bonnineau C, Geiszinger A, et al. Triclosan persistence through wastewater treatment plants and its potential toxic effects on river biofilms. Aquatic Toxicology. 2010;**100**(4):346-353. DOI: 10.1016/j.aquatox.2010.08.010

[63] Du H, Wang Q, Chen Y, Wu X, Jiang J, Zhao Y. Association between mixed exposure of phenols, parabens, phthalates and cognitive function in US elders. Journal of Affective Disorders. 2025;**382**:139-147. DOI: 10.1016/j.jad.2025.04.079

[64] Yen PL, How CM, Hsiu-Chuan LV. Early-life and chronic exposure to di(2-ethylhexyl) phthalate enhances amyloid-β toxicity associated with an autophagy-related gene in *Caenorhabditis elegans* Alzheimer's disease models. Chemosphere. 2021;**273**:128594. DOI: 10.1016/j.chemosphere.2020.128594

[65] Aldegunde-Louzao N, Lolo-Aira M, Herrero-Latorre C. Phthalate esters in different types of cosmetic products: A five-year quality control survey. Molecules. 2024;**29**(20):4823. DOI: 10.3390/molecules29204823

[66] Takacs-Vellai K, Vellai T, Puoti A, Passannante M, Wicky C, Streit A, et al. Inactivation of the autophagy gene bec-1 triggers apoptotic cell death in *C. Elegans*. Current Biology. 2005;**15**(16):1513-1517. DOI: 10.1016/j.cub.2005.07.035

[67] Borowska S, Brzóska MM. Metals in cosmetics: Implications for human health. Journal of Applied Toxicology. 2015;**35**(6):551-572. DOI: 10.1002/jat.3129

[68] Mold MJ, O'Farrell A, Morris B, Exley C. Aluminum and tau in neurofibrillary tangles in familial Alzheimer's disease. Journal of Alzheimer's Disease Reports. 2021;**5**(1):283-294. DOI: 10.3233/ADR-210011

[69] Pan B, Lu X, Han X, Huan J, Gao D, Cui S, et al. Mechanism by which aluminum regulates the abnormal phosphorylation of the tau protein in different cell lines. ACS Omega. 2021;**6**(47):31782-31796. DOI: 10.1021/acsomega.1c04434

[70] Rusina R, Matěj R, Kašparová L, Kukal J, Urban P. Higher aluminum concentration in Alzheimer's disease after box-cox data transformation. Neurotoxicity Research. 2011;**20**(4):329-333. DOI: 10.1007/s12640-011-9246-y

[71] McDonald JB, Dhakal S, Macreadie I. A toxic synergy between aluminium and amyloid beta in yeast. International Journal of Molecular Sciences. 2021;**22**(4):1835. DOI: 10.3390/ijms22041835

[72] Anghel L, Ciubară A, Nechita A, Nechita L, Manole C, Baroiu L, et al. Sleep disorders associated with neurodegenerative diseases. Diagnostics (Basel). 2023;**13**(18):2898. DOI: 10.3390/diagnostics13182898

[73] Wei Y, Wang Y, Lin CK, Yin K, Yang J, Shi L, et al. Associations between seasonal temperature and dementia-associated hospitalizations in New England. Environment International. 2019;**126**:228-233. DOI: 10.1016/j.envint.2018.12.054

[74] Culqui DR, Linares C, Ortiz C, Carmona R, Díaz J. Association between

environmental factors and emergency hospital admissions due to Alzheimer's disease in Madrid. The Science of the Total Environment. 2017;**592**:451-457. DOI: 10.1016/j.scitotenv.2017.03.089

[75] Delaney SW, Stegmuller A, Mork D, Mock L, Bell ML, Gill TM, et al. Extreme heat and hospitalization among older persons with Alzheimer disease and related dementias. JAMA Internal Medicine. 2025;**185**(4):412-421. DOI: 10.1001/jamainternmed.2024.7719

[76] Zhang R, Sun L, Jia A, Wang S, Guo Q, Wang Y, et al. Effect of heatwaves on mortality of Alzheimer's disease and other dementias among elderly aged 60 years and above in China, 2013-2020: A population-based study. The Lancet Regional Health. Western Pacific. 2024;**52**:101217. DOI: 10.1016/j.lanwpc.2024.101217

[77] Gong J, Part C, Hajat S. Current and future burdens of heat-related dementia hospital admissions in England. Environment International. 2022;**159**:107027. DOI: 10.1016/j.envint.2021.107027

[78] Brody GM. Hyperthermia and hypothermia in the elderly. Clinics in Geriatric Medicine. 1994;**10**(1):213-229

[79] Horwitz BA, Gabaldon AM, McDonald RB. Thermoregulation during aging. In: Hof PR, Mobbs CV, editors. Functional Neurobiology of Aging. San Diego (CA): Academic Press; 2001. pp. 839-854

[80] Fletcher PD, Downey LE, Golden HL, Clark CN, Slattery CF, Paterson RW, et al. Pain and temperature processing in dementia: A clinical and neuroanatomical analysis. Brain. 2015;**138**(Pt. 11):3360-3372. DOI: 10.1093/brain/awv276

[81] Thompson J, Vasefi M. Natural disaster-induced dementia and cognitive decline: A meta-analysis and systematic review. Social Science & Medicine. 2025;**371**:117898. DOI: 10.1016/j.socscimed.2025.117898

[82] Hikichi H, Aida J, Kondo K, Tsuboya T, Matsuyama Y, Subramanian SV, et al. Increased risk of dementia in the aftermath of the 2011 great East Japan earthquake and tsunami. Proceedings of the National Academy of Sciences of the United States of America. 2016;**113**(45):E6911-E6918. DOI: 10.1073/pnas.1607793113

[83] Norton MC, Fauth E, Clark CJ, Hatch D, Greene D, Pfister R, et al. Family member deaths across adulthood predict Alzheimer's disease risk: The Cache County study. International Journal of Geriatric Psychiatry. 2016;**31**(3):256-263. DOI: 10.1002/gps.4319

[84] Gibson A, Walsh J, Brown LM. A perfect storm: Challenges encountered by family caregivers of persons with Alzheimer's disease during natural disasters. Journal of Gerontological Social Work. 2018;**61**(7):775-789. DOI: 10.1080/01634372.2018.1474158

[85] Imam F, Saloner R, Vogel JW, Krish V, Abdel-Azim G, Ali M, et al. Global neurodegeneration proteomics consortium (GNPC). The global neurodegeneration proteomics consortium: Biomarker and drug target discovery for common neurodegenerative diseases and aging. Nature Medicine. 2025;**31**(8):2556-2566. DOI: 10.1038/s41591-025-03834-0

[86] Andrieu S, Bateman RJ, Bereczki E, et al. Harnessing artificial intelligence to transform Alzheimer's disease research. Nature Medicine. 2025;**31**(5):1384-1385. DOI: 10.1038/s41591-025-03632-8

Chapter 5

Protein Abundance Analysis in Amazonian Fish: Study of Mercury and Selenium Interaction Using Metalloproteomic Strategies

Izabela da Cunha Bataglioli, José Cavalcante Souza Vieira, Victor Diego Faria, Ronaldo de Almeida, Joyce Andrade da Silva, Luane B. Gonçalves Andrade, Felipe Dalmazzo Cirinêu, Luiz Fabrício Zara, Marília Afonso Rabelo Buzalaf, Jiri Adamec and Pedro de Magalhães Padilha

Abstract

The chapter reports the use of metalloproteomics strategies to identify the protein abundance in muscle tissue of *Psectrogaster amazonica* and *Raphiodon vulpinus* from Madeira River/Brazil exposed to mercury (Hg), with the aim of investigating possible Hg:Se interactions. Metalloproteomic results allowed the calculation of selenium values for health benefits (SeHBVs) that showed positive values for both fish species, suggesting that fish have Se reserves in their muscle tissue necessary to control the Hg toxic effects. Protein abundance analysis (PAA) showed that the few proteins and/or enzymes with up- and/or downregulated expression were expressed in the groups with higher Hg and Se concentrations. Therefore, it can be inferred that Se could be attenuating the Hg negative action on the functions of these proteins and/or enzymes through the formation of Se-Hg complexes in the structures of these macromolecules. The catalase, glutathione peroxidase and superoxide dismutase activity analysis, as well as that of lipoperoxides concentration, did not indicate that Hg concentrations present in muscle tissue of both fish species could trigger an oxidative stress state, corroborating with PAA results. The preliminary results obtained in the present chapter provide new insights into studies of the Se mitigating effect on the Hg toxicity in fish.

Keywords: Hg and Se in Amazonian fish, toxicity antagonism of Hg and Se, Hg and Se metallomics in fish, proteome damage, Hg and Se interaction new insights

1. Introduction

The toxic effects of mercurial species on humans and animals have been widely debated by the scientific community over the past four decades [1–3]. Several studies carried out in the Amazon region have found different concentrations of methylmercury in different species of fish, with the highest concentrations observed in predatory species. It is noteworthy that many of these species are frequently consumed by traditional populations in the Amazon [4–7].

Selenium (Se), a mineral with antioxidant properties, is important for the metabolic activity of humans and animals [8]. It is known that the presence of Se in the human diet can protect the brain against oxidative damage, can increase visual function and protect against cataracts and maculopathy, acts on the metabolism of thyroid hormones, in reproduction processes and other metabolic processes, as it is a component of more than 20 selenoproteins, with an emphasis on glutathione peroxidase (GPx) [9]. The capability of Se to mitigate the toxic effects of xenobiotics is a fundamental function of this micromineral. Several studies highlight the protective effects of Se against toxic elements, such as mercurial species, which have no biological function in organisms [10]. Hg-Se interaction mechanisms remain unclear. It is known that the protective effect of Se may be related to the formation of inert Hg-Se complexes; as the formation constant of Hg-Se association ($K_a = 10^{45}$) is greater than that of sulfur (S) (Hg-S, $K_a = 10^{39}$), Se can displace a large part of the Hg bound to the S-containing functional groups of proteins, which can reduce their toxicity [9]. Regarding fish, it is known that despite being an important source of protein in a healthy diet, fish—especially predatory fish—can contain significant levels of mercurial species [11]. The literature has reported that the molar excess of Se, which reflects an Se:Hg molar ratio greater than 1 in fish, could show that the Hg concentration does not present toxic effects, and the consumption of fish can therefore be safe [11, 12].

Metallomics, a recent line of research, makes it possible to investigate the interactions and functional connections between genes, metabolites, proteins, and other biomolecules of an organism with metallic species [13]. The aim of metallomics is to clarify the biological role of metallic species and/or metalloids that bind to biomolecules and the function thereof in an organism [14, 15]. In this context, metallomics can provide new insights to elucidate the attenuating effect of Se in relation to Hg toxicity in fish.

Accordingly, this manuscript reports the obtained results using metallomic strategies (the association of graphite furnace atomic absorption spectrometry [GFAAS] techniques with *Shotgun*—LC-MS/MS) in a study on the mitigating effect of Se on Hg toxicity in the organism of *P. amazonica* (a non-carnivorous species) and *R. vulpinus* (a carnivorous species) from the Jirau region along the Madeira River in the state of Rondonia in the Brazilian Amazon. In the last few decades, the Madeira River has been impacted by mercury due to gold mining activities [16]. The *P. amazonica* and *R. vulpinus* species were chosen because they are primarily consumed by the traditional population of the Brazilian Amazon [17, 18].

2. Material and methods

2.1 Fish collection and sample processing

The Chico Mendes Institute for Biodiversity Conservation and Authorization and Information System on Biodiversity (ICMBio; Ref. SISBIO 43890-1) and the Committee on Ethics in the Use of Animals (CEUA), protocol number n° 0316/2023, authorized this research. Eight individuals of the species *P. amazonica* (branquinha) with a medium size of 17 ± 2 cm and 350 ± 21 g and eight individuals of the species *R. vulpinus* (cachorra) with a medium size of 26 ± 3 cm and 620 ± 52 g were captured in the area of the Jirau Hydroelectric Plant reservoir on the Madeira River in the Rondonia state of Brazil. The collection points were: (a) (S 09°47′18.3″; W 065°31′12.4″); (b) (S 09°41′0.06″; WE 064°58′43.9″); and (c) (S 09°16′12.8″; W 064°41′14″). The fish were captured by a team of biologists from ESBR Company (Brazil's Sustainable Energy), using nets made of mesh measuring 1.5 cm × 10 cm from one side to the other. The fish were euthanized on site soon after capture by myelotomy followed by cranial drilling. The muscle tissue samples were then removed and immediately transferred to Falcon tubes and stored in liquid nitrogen. The samples were subsequently transported to the Bioanalytical and Metalloproteomic Laboratory (LBM) of the Institute of Biosciences—UNESP, where they were stored in a freezer at −80°C until metalloproteomic and oxidative-stress analyses were performed.

2.2 Hg and Se determinations

The analysis of Hg_T and Se_T in muscle tissue samples and pellets was performed using GFAAS following the method outlined by Silva et al. [19] and Moraes et al. [20]. In brief, the procedure entails the mineralization of samples using a mixture of concentrated sulfuric acid and 30% (m/m) hydrogen peroxide in an ultrasound-assisted heating bath. The resulting acid extracts were then adjusted to a final volume of 5.00 mL in volumetric flasks. To maintain the thermal stabilization of Hg and Se during atomization, a combination of tungsten as a permanent chemical modifier and zirconium as chemical modifier co-injected with the sample into the graphite tube, were employed. The analyses were conducted using a SHIMADZU AA-6800 atomic absorption spectrometer, which is equipped with a background corrector featuring a self-reverse system and a deuterium lamp, as well as a pyrolytic graphite tube with an integrated platform and an AS6100 automatic sampler. All determinations of Hg_T and Se_T were validated by analyzing the DORM 4 certified reference material produced by the National Research Council of Canada. Based on the findings from the Hg_T and Se_T determinations in muscle tissue samples, the ratios of Hg:Se and Se:Hg were calculated, along with the Se values associated with health benefits (SeHBVs) [12].

2.3 Protein abundance analysis by shotgun: LC-MS/MS

The process outlined by Bataglioli et al. [21] was followed to extract the protein fraction from muscle samples using Tris-HCl buffer pH 8.80 under denaturing conditions for protein abundance analysis (PAA). Following successive centrifugation operations at 12,000xg for 30 minutes at 4°C, the transparent protein extracts were obtained. The total protein concentration was then calculated to normalize the protein masses at 50 μg in all extracts from eight fish with lower HgT and SeT concentrations (i.e., the control group) and eight fish with higher HgT and SeT concentrations (i.e., experimental groups). A PAA in the muscle proteome of the *P. amazonica* and *R. vulpinus* species was performed by *Shotgun*—LC-MS/MS according to the procedures already described by Bittencourt et al. [21]. Peptide identifications were performed on a nanoACQUITY UPLC-Xevo QT of MS system (Waters, Manchester, UK). The nanoACQUITY UPLC® was equipped with a nanoACQUITY HSS T3 reversed-phase analytical column (75 μm × 150 mm, 1.8 μm particle size). The Xevo® G2 Q-TOF mass spectrometer was operated in nanoelectrospray positive ion mode, and data were collected using the mean squared-error method at high energy (19–45 V), which allows data acquisition of both precursor and fragment ions in a single injection. The source conditions included 2.5 kV capillary voltage, 30.0 V sample cone, 5.0 V extraction cone, and 80°C temperature. Data were acquired over 70 minutes, scanning in the range of 50–2000 Da. The lockspray, which was used to ensure accuracy and reproducibility, was operated with a solution of [Glu1] fibrinopeptide (1 pmol/μL), with a flow rate of 1 μL/min, as a reference ion in positive mode at m/z 785.8427. The mass spectrometry raw data files were uploaded to Progenesis QI for Proteomics v4.0 (Nonlinear Dynamics, Waters, and Newcastle upon Tyne, UK) to perform a quantitative analysis [22]. For alignment, a sample result was automatically selected as a reference. The remaining results were aligned with the reference with an alignment score greater than 80%, and peak picking was performed using the automatic sensitivity method. Peak intensities were then normalized by calculating abundance ratios relative to a reference. The peak list was searched in the UniProtKB/Swiss-Prot database using Otophysi class data and the Mascot 2.6 software (Matrix Science, London, UK). Trypsin was the specified enzyme, and one missed cleavage was allowed. Cysteine carbamidomethylation was defined as a fixed modification and methionine oxidation as a variable modification. A precursor mass tolerance of 10 ppm and a fragment ion tolerance of 0.01 Da were applied; a false discovery rate of 1% was considered [21, 22].

2.4 Parameter analysis related to oxidative stress

A parameter analysis related to oxidative stress was conducted on homogenates after extraction with 0.01 mol L^{-1} phosphate buffer with pH 7.00 in an OMNI/Analytical cell disruptor. For this analysis, 0.20 g of muscle tissue samples from each of the individuals of the lower C_{Hg} and Se groups and the higher C_{Hg} and Se groups of *P. amazonica* and *R. vulpinus* species (i.e., the biological replicates) were used. The suspensions obtained were centrifuged at 12,000xg for 30 minutes at 4°C, and transparent supernatants were obtained. Lipid lipoperoxidation (LPO), GPx, catalase (CAT), and superoxide dismutase (SOD) activities were determined using methodologies already consolidated and published in the extant literature. In case, the GPx activity was indirectly determined by a previously described method [23] based on the oxidation of reduced GSH. CAT activity was determined by ultraviolet spectrophotometry as previously described [24]; SOD activity was determined according to a reported protocol [25]; and the LPO marker was determined using the Jiang procedure [26] based on the oxidation of Fe^{2+} to Fe^{3+} ions by lipoperoxide at an acidic pH in the presence of a xylenol orange metallochromic indicator.

2.5 Statistical analysis

The results of Hg and Se determinations were expressed as the mean ± standard deviation, and checked whether they were in agreement with the values of the certified reference material using the Student's t test and an F test and SAS Version 8 statistical software. The significance level considered was 5% ($p < 0.05$) [27, 28]. In relation to data from the CAT, SOD, GPx activity analysis, and the LPO concentrations, the Spearman Correlation test was used to evaluate the correlation of these parameters with the Hg_T and Se_T concentrations [29]. The PAA data were analyzed using the nanoAcquity UPLC Xevo QTof MS and Protein Lynx Global Server software (version 2.5). For this, a relative quantification using non-conflicting peptides was selected to quantify the protein or proteins; to be considered with relative abundance variation, it should be identified and quantified using at least two unique peptides and present a p-value <0.05 (i.e., down-regulated proteins) and a 1-p value >0.95 (i.e., upregulated proteins) [21, 22].

3. Results and discussion

3.1 Hg and Se determinations

Hg_T and Se_T concentrations were determined in eight muscle tissue samples and four protein pellet pools derived from *P. amazonica* and *R. vulpinus*. For muscle tissue, approximately 100 mg from each of eight individual fish samples were mineralized. Hg_T and Se_T determinations were then performed using Graphite Furnace Atomic Absorption Spectrometry (GFAAS), following the procedures detailed by Silva et al. [19] and Moraes et al. [20]. In relation to protein pellets, the extraction and precipitation of the protein fraction was carried out in four pools of muscle tissue samples—in this case, a pool with samples from individuals with the highest concentration of Hg_T and Se_T and a pool with samples from individuals with the highest concentration of Hg_T and $Se_{T,}$ for the two species of fish, making a total of four pools. The results obtained are summarized in **Figure 1**.

Figure 1 (Graphics 1–4) illustrates the separation of individuals from both *P. amazonica* and *R. vulpinus* into two distinct groups based on Hg_T and Se_T concentrations: a low-concentration group and a high-concentration group. For *P. amazonica*, individuals in groups 1, 3, 6, and 7 (Graphics 1 and 2) exhibited lower mean C_{HgT} (6.91 ± 0.117.6 4 ± 0.14 μg kg^{-1}) and C_{SeT} (10.71 ± 0.16 μg kg^{-1} to 11.84 ± 0.21 μg kg^{-1}). This collective was designated as $PaHgSe_1$ (low C_{HgT} and C_{SeT}). Conversely, individuals from groups 2, 4, 5, and 8 of *P. amazonica* (Graphics 1 and 2) showed significantly higher mean C_{HgT} (34.46 ± 0.17 μg kg^{-1} to 36.15 ± 0.47 μg kg^{-1}) and C_{SeT} (42.04 ± 0.63 μg kg^{-1} to 44.10 ± 0.83 μg kg^{-1}), forming the PaHgSe2 group high C_{HgT} and C_{SeT}. Similarly, for *R. vulpinus*, C_{HgT} and C_{SeT} mean values allowed for the creation of two groups. Individuals in groups 1, 3, 4, and 7 (Graphics 3 and 4) constituted RvHgSe 1, presenting lower mean C_{HgT} (25.65 ± 0.45 μg kg^{-1} to 32.46 ± 0.54 μg kg^{-1} and C_{SeT} (41.81 ± 0.78 μg kg^{-1} to 52.30 ± 0.89 μg kg^{-1}). The second group, $RvHgSe_2$, comprising individuals 2, 5, 6, and 8 (Graphics 3 and 4), exhibited the highest mean C_{HgT} (51.70 ± 0.93 μg kg^{-1} to 55.48 ± 0.99 μg kg^{-1}) and C_{SeT} (62.20 ± 1.07 μg kg^{-1} to 66.44 ± 1.13 μg kg^{-1}).

The determined C_{HgT} *and* C_{SeT} values facilitated the calculation of Hg:Se and Se:Hg molar ratios for all four individual groups of *P. amazonica* and *R. vulpinus*. The average molar ratios were as follows [12, 30]:

- $PaHgSe_1$ (*P. amazonica* with low C_{HgT} and C_{SeT}): Hg:Se = 0.26; Se:Hg = 3.9
- $PaHgSe_2$ (*P. amazonica* with high C_{HgT} and C_{SeT}): Hg:Se = 0.32; Se:Hg = 2.9
- $Rv\text{-}HgSe_1$ (*R. vulpinus* with low C_{HgT} and C_{SeT}): Hg:Se = 0.26; Se:Hg = 3.8
- $RvHgSe_2$ (*R. vulpinus* with high C_{HgT} and C_{SeT}): Hg:Se = 0.33; Se:Hg = 3.0

From these molar ratios, the Selenium health benefit value (SeHBV) was calculated using Eq. 1 [31, 32]:

$$SeHBV = [Se : Hg \times Se(\mu mol\, kg^{-1})] - [Hg : Se \times Se(\mu mol\, kg^{-1})] \qquad (1)$$

- $PaHgSe_1$: SeHBV = 0.54

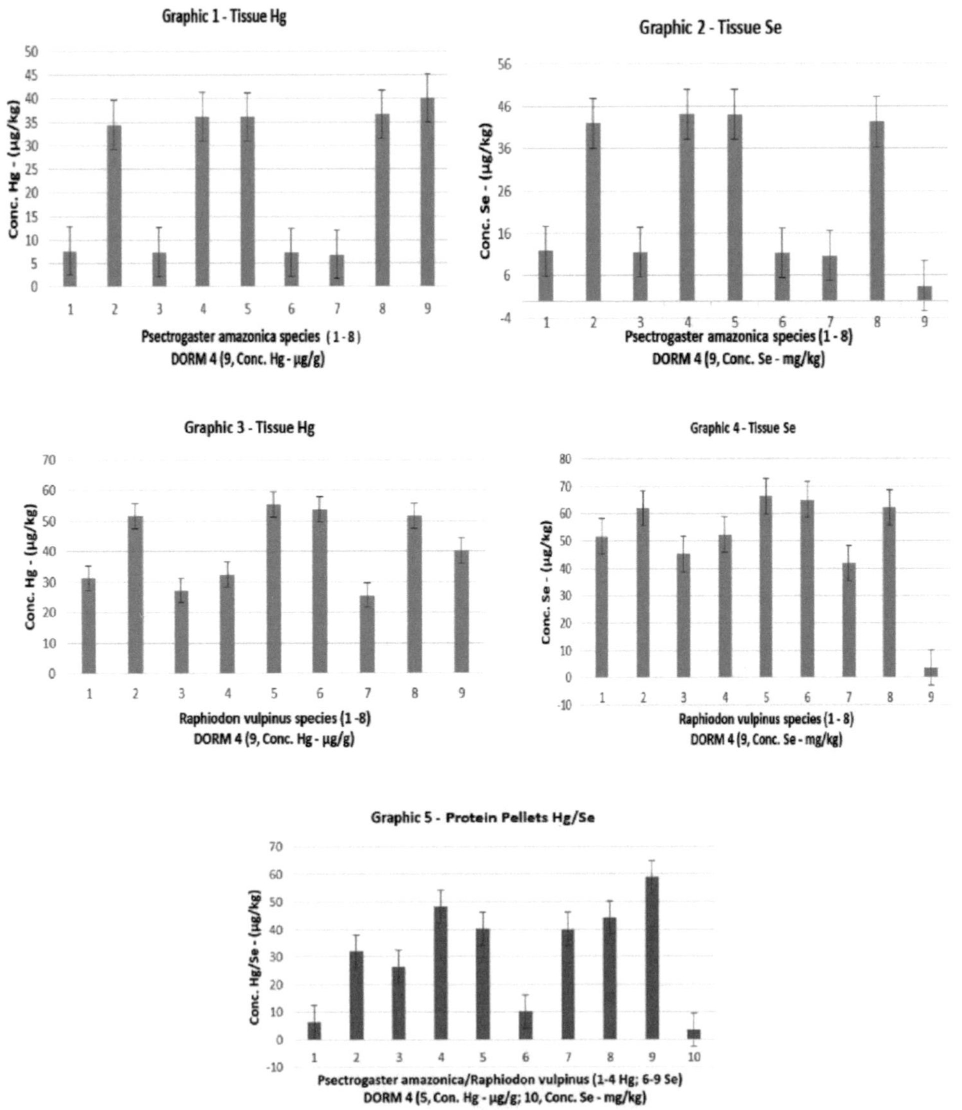

Figure 1.

Total Hg and Se concentrations in muscle, protein pellets of tissue samples from P. amazonica and R. vulpinus species, and DORM 4 (CRM) (Graphic 1: bars 1, 3, 6, and 7: P. amazonica *with lower $[Hg_{total}]$; bars 2, 4, 5, and 8:* P. amazonica *species with higher $[Hg_{total}]$; bar 9: C_{Hg}(μg/100 g), DORM 4; Graphic 2: bars 1, 3, 6, and 7:* P. amazonica *with lower $[Se_{total}]$; bar 2, 4. 5, and 8:* P. amazonica *with higher $[Se_{total}]$; bar 9: C_{Se}(mg/kg), DORM 4; Graphic 3: bars 1, 3, 4, and 7:* R. vulpinus *with lower $[Hg_{total}]$; bars 2, 5, 6, and 8:* R. vulpinus *with higher $[Hg_{total}]$; bar 9: C_{Hg}(μg/100 g), DORM 4; Graphic 4: bars 1, 3, 4, and 7:* R. vulpinus *with lower $[Se_{total}]$; bars 2, 5, 6, and 8:* R. vulpinus *with higher $[Se_{total}]$; bar 9: C_{Se}(mg/kg); DORM 4; Graphic 5: bars 1 and 6:* pool *of* P. amazonica *with lower $[Hg_{total}]$ and $[Se_{total}]$; bars 2 and 7: pool of* P. amazonica *species with higher $[Hg_{total}]$ and $[Se_{total}]$; bars 3 and 8:* pool *of* R. vulpinus *with lower $[Hg_{total}]$ and $[Se_{total}]$; bars 4 and 9:* pool *of* R. vulpinus *with higher $[Hg_{total}]$ and $[Se_{total}]$; bar 5: C_{Hg}(μg/100 g), bar 10: C_{Se}(mg/kg), DORM 4).*

- $PaHgSe_2$: SeHBV = 1.7
- $RvHgSe_1$: SeHBV = 2.3
- $RvHgSe_2$: SeHBV = 2.3

Notably, the calculated Se:Hg molar ratios were consistently greater than 1 for both fish species. Furthermore, all calculated SeHBV values were positive; specifically, SeHBV values for the Pa-HgSe 2 group were greater than 1, and for both groups of *R. vulpinus*, values were also positive and greater than 1. These findings suggest that the mercury concentrations observed in both the non-carnivorous *P. amazonica* and the carnivorous *R. vulpinus* species pose a low health risk [7]. This is further supported by the presence of sufficient selenium reserves (acting as a soft base) within the muscle tissue of both species, which can readily complex with mercury species (acting as soft acids) to form stable Se-Hg complexes [33]. Based on the C_{HgT} and C_{SeT} determinations in muscle tissues of *P. amazonica* and *R. vulpinus*, protein fractions were extracted from muscle tissue pools corresponding to the $PaHgSe_1$, $PaHgSe_2$, $RvHgSe_1$, and $RvHgSe_2$ groups. Total mercury and selenium determinations were subsequently performed on the respective protein pellets using GFAAS. The results are summarized in **Figure 1** (Graphic 5). Analysis of these results revealed that the Hg_T and Se_T concentrations in the protein pellets from $PaHgSe_1$, $PaHgSe_2$, $RvHgSe_1$, and $RvHgSe_2$ groups were consistent with the initial muscle tissue determinations. Specifically, C_{HgT} and C_{SeT} were higher in the $PaHgSe_2$ and $RvHgSe_2$ groups (Graphic 5: bars 2, 4, 7, and 9) compared to the $PaHgSe_1$ and $RvHgSe_1$ groups (Graphic 5: bars 1, 3, 6, and 8). This consistency validates the use of individuals from the $PaHgSe_1$ and $RvHgSe_1$ groups (control groups) and the $PaHgSe_2$ and $RvHgSe_2$ groups as biological replicates for subsequent protein abundance analysis (PAA) of the muscle proteome in both *P. amazonica* and *R. vulpinus*. Finally, method robustness was confirmed by the Hg_T and Se_T determinations in the certified reference material DORM 4 (fish protein). A recovery percentage of approximately 98% and a relative standard deviation of less than 2 were achieved, demonstrating the reliability of the analytical procedure [16].

3.2 PAA in muscle proteome of the *P. amazonica* and *R. vulpinus* species

The fractionation and characterization experiments and PAA in muscle proteome of the *P. amazonica* and *R. vulpinus* species were carried out after the proteolytic cleavage procedures of the protein extracts, according to the procedure described in *Item 2.3*. PAA were performed by comparing the $PaHgSe_1$ and $RvHgSe_1$ groups (i.e., lower C_{HgSe}) with the $PaHgSe_2$ and $RvHgSe_2$ groups (i.e., higher C_{HgSe}) of the two fish species, based on the results obtained in the determinations of selenium and mercury and in the C_{SeT} and C_{HgT} values, as well as the SeHBV that was calculated. The obtained results are summarized in **Tables 1** and **2**. The results regarding the analysis of proteins/enzymes that did not show significant relative abundance variance are shown in Table S1 (Supplementary Information).

It was observed that a few proteins showed *up* or *downregulation* in the muscle proteome of both fish species. In this case, six proteins had downregulation and 10 had *upregulation* in the muscle proteome of *P. amazonica*, and only one protein presented *downregulation* and two *upregulation* in the muscle proteome of *R. vulpinus* species. Regarding the proteins that were *Unique*, eight proteins were only expressed in the $PaHgSe_2$ group of the muscle proteome of the *P. amazonica,* and ten in the $RvHgSe_2$ group of the *R. vulpinus*. The proteins and/or enzymes that were *Unique* and/or with different expressions will be discussed next to investigate a possible correlation with the C_{HgT} and C_{SeT} determined in the $PaHgSe_2$ and $RvHgSe_2$ groups.

Concerning proteins, the literature reports that the Hemoglobin subunits (Hbs) (the proteins involved in oxygen transport from the gills to peripheral tissues in fish); the Histone/isoforms (i.e., the proteins that act in the regulation of DNA

Access	Description	Score	
	***Unique* Proteins**		**Groups**
A8WGB	Collagen and calcium-binding EGF domain-containing protein 1	104,97	$PaHgSe_2$
P02018	Hemoglobin subunit alpha	318,92	$PaHgSe_2$
O13163	Hemoglobin subunit beta	216,59	$PaHgSe_2$
Q5BJA5	Histone H2B 1/2	428,6	$PaHgSe_2$
Q6PC60	Histone H2B 3	428,6	$PaHgSe_2$
Q9W7K5	L-lactate dehydrogenase A chain	531,76	$PaHgSe_2$
Q9PVK4	L-lactate dehydrogenase B-A chain	390,24	$PaHgSe_2$
Q6DGK2	L-lactate dehydrogenase B-B chain	150,28	$PaHgSe_2$
	***Downregulated* proteins**		**PaHgSe2 x PaHgSe1**
P83751	Actin_ cytoplasmic 1	233,91	0
Q7ZVF9	Actin_ cytoplasmic 2	233,91	0
Q9PVK4	L-lactate dehydrogenase B-A chain	121.18	0.01
Q5XJ10	Glyceraldehyde-3-phosphate dehydrogenase	343.5	0
Q1MTI4	Triosephosphate isomerase A	178.69	0
Q90XG0	Triosephosphate isomerase B	178.69	0
	***Upregulated* proteins**		**PaHgSe2 x PaHgSe1**
Q90339	Myosin heavy chain_ fast skeletal muscle	180,57	1
P13104	Tropomyosin alpha-1 chain	561,4	1
Q9I8V0	Parvalbumin-2	173.34	1
P02618	Parvalbumin beta	659.38	1
O93409	Myosin regulatory light chain 2_ skeletal muscle isoform A	751.23	1
P53479	Actin_ alpha skeletal muscle	2193.15	1
P09227	Parvalbumin alpha	173.34	1
Q90339	Myosin heavy chain_ fast skeletal muscle	1264.44	1
Q6P0G6	Myosin_ light chain 1_ alkali; skeletal_ fast	638.78	1
P12115	Adenylate kinase isoenzyme 1	169.24	1

Table 1.
Proteins identified in the muscle tissue of P. amazonica *species ($PaHgSe_2$ x $PaHgSe_1$). Unique proteins were expressed only in the group pool with the highest C_{HgT} and C_{SeT} ($PaHgSe_2$).*

transcription); were identified in Hg-linked protein spots (C_{Hg} in protein spots: 2–20 mg kg^{-1}) in the muscle, liver, and kidney proteomes of fish from the Amazon [34–37]. The collagen protein and the calcium-binding EGF domain-containing protein 1 (CCBE1) participate in lymphangioblast budding and angiogenic sprouting of the venous endothelium during embryogenesis [34, 38]; these were only expressed in the $PaHgSe_2$ and $RvHgSe_2$ groups. While the extant literature does not report Hg binding in CCBE1 structures, CCBE1 also has a FASTA sequence with cysteine and methionine residues, which are amino acids that have thiol and thioether groups,

Access	Description	Score	
	***Unique* Proteins**		**Groups**
Q32LQ4	Betaine--homocysteine S-methyltransferase 1	148,44	$RvHgSe_2$
P82316	Hemoglobin cathodic subunit beta	230,72	$RvHgSe_2$
P02018	Hemoglobin subunit alpha	1592,19	$RvHgSe_2$
Q90486	Hemoglobin subunit beta-1	1581,28	$RvHgSe_2$
Q90485	Hemoglobin subunit beta-2	904,89	$RvHgSe_2$
P85312	Hemoglobin subunit beta-A (Fragment)	824,97	$RvHgSe_2$
P02139	Hemoglobin subunit beta-A/B	1501,36	$RvHgSe_2$
P85313	Hemoglobin subunit beta-B (Fragment)	824,97	$RvHgSe_2$
Q4KMC8	Fructose-bisphosphate aldolase C-A	172,71	$RvHgSe_2$
	***Downregulated* proteins**		**RvHgSe2 x RvHgSe1**
Q5XJ10	Glyceraldehyde-3-phosphate dehydrogenase	872,52	0
	***Upregulated* proteins**		**RvHgSe2 x RvHgSe1**
O93409	Myosin regulatory light chain 2_ skeletal muscle isoform A	1069,32	1
Q90339	Myosin heavy chain_ fast skeletal muscle	658.15	1

Table 2.
Proteins identified in the muscle tissue of R. vulpinus *species ($RvHgSe_2$ × $RvHgSe_1$. Unique proteins were expressed only in the group pool with the highest C_{HgT} and C_{SeT} ($RvHgSe_2$).*

respectively (i.e., soft bases) [33]. As such, Hg and Se coordination (i.e., soft acids) may occur in the CCBE1 structure. A metalloproteomic study by Almeida et al. [39] reported the identification of Hb beta 1, 2, and alpha ½-subunits in Hg-linked protein spots in the renal proteome of rats exposed to mercuric chloride (C_{Hg} in protein spots: 84–138 mg kg^{-1}). The authors posited that the PAA variance indicated that the beta 1, 2, and alpha ½-subunits of Hb showed *downregulation*, which could qualify the Hb subunits as possible biomarkers of exposure to the Hg species. In the same study [39], the authors reported that PAA indicated that H3.1 and H3.3 were only expressed in the control group of rats exposed to mercuric chloride ($HgCl_2$); this result corroborates data from a metalloproteomic study by Bittarello et al. [35], who examined kidney tissue from the *Colossoma macropomum* species from the Amazon River, which reports the identification of Histone H4 in Hg-linked protein spots (C_{Hg} = 5.85 mg kg^{-1}).

The L-lactate dehydrogenase (LDH) enzyme and isoform (i.e., the enzyme that acts in converting pyruvate to lactate process in carbohydrate and carboxylic metabolic acids); betaine-homocysteine S-methyltransferase (BHMT) (i.e., the enzyme that catalyzes the betaine conversion and homocysteine to dimethylglycine and methionine, respectively); and fructose-bisphosphate aldolase C-A (ALDOCA) (i.e., the enzyme that presents Zn^{2+} specific domains in its side chains and acts in gluconeogenesis reactions) also showed expression only in the $PaHgSe_2$ and $RvHgSe_2$ groups [34].

The literature further reports that LDH and isoforms, BHMT, and ALDOCA were identified in Hg-linked protein spots (C_{Hg} in protein spots: ranging from 3 to 160 mg kg^{-1}) in the muscle, liver, and kidney proteomes from Amazon fish

[35, 40–43]. These authors explained that the binding of Hg species in three enzyme structures directly affects the biological activities thereof. Since PAA was not carried out to identify whether there was impairment in the enzymes' expression in respective proteomes, however, the robustness of these conclusions was compromised. The LDH/isoforms, BHMT, and ALDOCA have cysteine and methionine residues in the FASTA sequences and amino acids that have thiol and thioether groups (i.e., soft bases), respectively. Thiol and thioether groups can form stable bonds with Hg and Se species (i.e., soft acids) [33, 35, 39]. BHMT and ALDOCA also have specific domains for Zn^{2+} ions; when this happens, Hg and Se species could displace Zn^{2+} from these domains, thereby binding to these enzyme structures [41, 44]. Regarding the BHMT enzyme, it is noteworthy that metalloproteomic study with rats exposed to $HgCl_2$ using 2D PAGE-GFAAS-LC-MS/MS, reported that BHMT was only expressed in Hg-linked protein spots (C_{Hg} = 15.40 mg kg^{-1}) of the liver proteome of rats exposed to $HgCl_2$ [43]. This finding corroborates data reported in the present study and in the study by Queiroz et al. 2019 [44] cited above.

This study, PAA results revealed that Hbs subunits, histone/isoforms, and the enzymes LDH/isoforms, BHMT, and ALDOCA were expressed as unique proteins/enzymes in the muscle proteome of *P. amazonica* ($PaHgSe_2$ group) and *R. vulpinus* ($RvHgSe_2$ group). $PaHgSe_2$ and $RvHgSe_2$ groups exhibited higher total mercury (C_{HgT}) and total selenium (C_{SeT}) concentrations in both muscle tissue and protein pellets, with C_{SeT} levels exceeding to C_{HgT}, resulting in positive SeHBVs. This suggests that *P. amazonica* and *R. vulpinus* possess Se reserves in their muscle tissue, enabling them to counteract the toxic effects of Hg [12, 31, 32]. The presence of Se likely leads to the formation of *metal-binding proteins* (*MBPs*), specifically involving complexes such as [SeHg]-Hbs, [SeHg]-Histones, [SeHg]-CCBE1, [SeHg]-LDH/isoforms, [SeHg]-BHMT, and [SeHg]-ALDOCA. The binding of the [SeHg]-complex (a soft acid) to these protein/enzyme structures is likely facilitated by thiol (R-SH) and/or thioether groups (soft bases) on cysteine and methionine residues within their FASTA sequences, as previously discussed [33, 34, 42]. Consequently, the [SeHg]-MBPs were exclusively expressed in the $PaHgSe_2$ and $RvHgSe_2$ groups, which exhibited elevated C_{SeT} and C_{HgT} levels.

Regarding the *upregulation* and/or *downregulation* results (**Tables 1** and **2**), only seven proteins and 12 proteins and/or enzymes showed a decrease and/or increase in expression in the $PaHgSe_2$ and $RvHgSe_2$ groups, respectively. It is noteworthy that the $PaHgSe_1$ group (group of non-predator species, which presented lower concentrations of Hg and Se in relation to $RvHgSe_1$ group from predator species), also presented a greater number of proteins and/or enzymes with up and/or downregulation; this may indicates that this effect may not be related to the binding of Se and Hg species in the structures of these proteins and/or enzymes. When analyzing the results in **Tables 1** and **2**, it is therefore possible to highlight the actin (*actbb and acta1*) and parvalbumin isoforms (*pvalb2, pvalbβ, and pavalbα*), the enzyme glyceraldehyde-3-phosphate dehydrogenase (*gapdh*), and triosephosphate isomerase isoforms (*tpi1a* and *tpi1b*), which were expressed with *up-* or *downregulation* in the muscle proteome of the $PaHgSe_2$ group.

Metalloproteomic studies with *Semaprochilodus* spp. and *Arapaima gigas* from the Amazon region reported the identification of actbb and acta1 isoforms and pvalb2, pvalbα, and pavalbβ isoforms in Hg-linked protein spots of the muscle and liver proteomes of these fish [40, 41]. The gapdh enzyme and the tpi1a and tpi1b isoforms were identified in Hg-linked protein spots in the muscle and liver proteomes of *Brachyplatystoma rousseauxii*, *Mylossoma sp.*, *Myleus sp.*, *Prochilodus nigricans*, and *Cichla sp.*—which are species of fish from the Amazon region—and also through metalloproteomic strategies [40, 45]. However, these papers did not perform PAA to investigate whether actbb and acta; pvalb2, pvalbα, and pavalbβ; tpi1a and tpi1b; and gapdh showed expression differences, which limited the discussion of results.

The myosin isoforms, the tropomyosin alpha 1 chain (tpma), and adenylate kinase isoenzyme 1 (ak1) were expressed with *upregulation* primarily in the PaHgSe group. To date, the literature does not report studies related to Hg or Se species associated with myosin, tpma, or ak1. As these proteins/enzymes were expressed with upregulation in higher quantities in *P. amazonica* (non-predator species) muscle proteome, the species that presented lower C_{Se} and C_{Hg}, the expression increase may not be related to the Se and Hg concentrations in the fish muscle tissue. It stands out that only two myosin isoforms were expressed with *upregulation* and gapdh enzyme was expressed with *downregulation* in the RvHgSe group (predator species with higher concentration of Hg and Se), o can reinforce the indication of the non-relationship of Se an Hg concentrations to the differences in abundance variance *up/down* of proteins/enzymes shown in **Tables 1** and **2**.

3.3 Analysis of parameters related to oxidative stress

The results obtained for CAT, GPx, and SOD activity, the LPO activity, and the LPO concentration are summarized in **Figure 2** and **Table 3**. The CAT, GPx, and SOD activities and the LPO concentration were carried out with the aim of investigating whether Hg concentrations present in the organisms of the *P. amazonica* and *R. vulpinus* species could trigger an oxidative stress state.

Analysis of **Figure 2** suggests no apparent correlation between CHgT and CSeT and the activities of SOD, CAT, and GPx enzymes, or LPO concentration. This held true for both *P. amazonica* and *R. vulpinus*, regardless of whether individuals exhibited lower (red bars) or higher (blue bars) concentrations of Se and Hg. Specifically, maximum and minimum values for CAT, SOD, and GPx activities, as well as LPO concentrations, were observed across individuals with varying Hg and/or Se levels. The Spearman correlation coefficient (CCSp) values, calculated by correlating the lowest CHgT and CSeT with these enzymatic activities and LPO concentration (as shown in **Table 3**), followed the same behavior. Seven positive CCSp values ranging from 0.59 to 0.89, and nine negative CCSp values ranging from −0.54 to −0.98. Notably, most of these CCSp values (both positive and negative) were not statistically significant ($p \geq 0.05$). Analysis of LPO concentrations revealed a consistent pattern across both fish species: groups with lower total mercury (C_{HgT}) and total selenium (C_{SeT}) exhibited significant negative correlations (CCSp.−, $p < 0.05$). Conversely, LPO correlations were not significant in groups with higher C_{HgT} and C_{SeT}. For the CAT activity, only *R. vulpinus* groups with lower C_{HgT} and C_{SeT} showed negative correlations (CCSp.−); all other CAT correlations in both species were not significant. The results for SOD activity were more varied. In *P. amazonica*, we found significant positive correlations (CCSp.+) in groups with lower C_{SeT}, but no significant correlation in groups with lower C_{HgT}. For *R. vulpinus*, significant negative correlations (CCSp.−) were observed in groups with lower C_{HgT} and C_{SeT}, though these correlations became non-significant at higher C_{HgT} and C_{SeT} levels. Lastly, for GPx activity in *P. amazonica*, groups with lower C_{HgT} and C_{SeT} displayed significant positive correlations (CCSp.+), while correlations were not significant in groups with higher C_{HgT} and C_{SeT}. Notably, in *R. vulpinus*, GPx activity exhibited significant positive Spearman correlation coefficients (CCSp.+) for

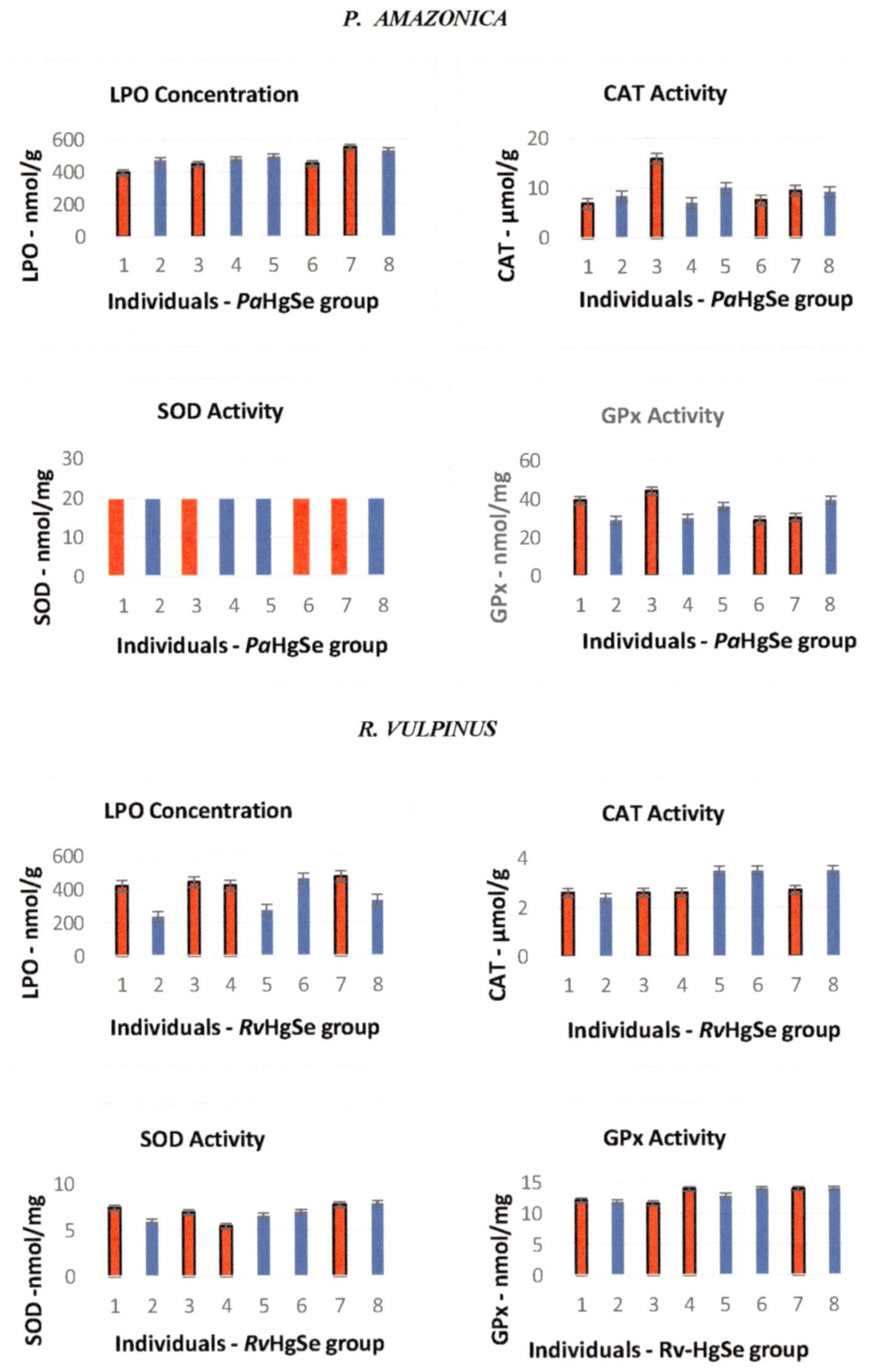

Figure 2.
Activity of SOD, CAT, and GPx enzymes, and LPO concentration were determined in the muscle tissue of "individuals" of P. amazonica *and* R. vulpinus *species.*

Variables	LPO CCSp.	CAT CCSp.	SOD CCSp.	GPx CCSp.
P. amazonica	—	—	—	—
Group with <C_{HgT}	−0.9840*	−0.04105ND	−0.5412*	0.6137*
Group with >C_{HgT}	−0.2419ND	−0.1160ND	0.4781ND	−0,06230ND
Group with <C_{SeT}	−0.9829*	−0.04270ND	0.7915*	0.6310*
Group with >C_{SeT}	−0.2424ND	−0.1142ND	0.5963*	−0.06270ND
R. vulpinus	—	—	—	—
Group with <C_{HgT}	−0.9413*	−0.7287*	−0.6072*	0.4106ND
Group with >C_{HgT}	−0.4641ND	0.4074ND	−0.1865ND	0.7909*
Group with <C_{SeT}	−0.9625*	−0.7835*	−0.6168*	0.5275*
Group with >C_{SeT}	−0.2537ND	0.4233ND	−0.3355ND	0.8906*

CCSp. – Spearman correlation coefficient. *Significant ($p < 0.05$).*
ND*Non-significant ($p \geq 0.05$).*

Table 3.
Spearman's correlation coefficient calculated in relation to C_{HgT} and C_{SeT}, and the activities of the enzymes CAT, SOD and GPx, and LPO concentration in the muscle tissue of P. amazonica *and* R. vulpinus.

groups with higher C_{HgT}, as well as both lower and higher C_{SeT}. These findings contrast with those reported by Bittarello et al. [35], who studied *Plagioscion squamosissimus* (carnivorous) and *Colossoma macropomum* (omnivorous) from the Brazilian Amazon. They observed a trend toward increased GPx activity and lipid peroxidation (LPO) concentration in the liver tissue of *P. squamosissimus*, which also had higher C_{HgT}. However, their calculated CCSp values indicated a negative correlation between GPx activity and C_{HgT} (−0.7040, for C_{HgT} = 279 ± 4.41μgkg − 1). This is contrary to our current study, which found a positive correlation. Bittarello et al. [35] proposed that the inhibition of GPx by mercury could be linked to a mercury-selenol interaction. However, they did not measure selenium levels in the fish liver tissue samples, which would have provided stronger support for their conclusions.

In this study, we observed a positive correlation between GPx activities and C_{HgT} in *R. vulpinus*, a species known to accumulate higher levels of mercury. Interestingly, we also found a positive correlation with C_{SeT}, with C_{SeT} being higher than C_{HgT}. The selenium measurements allowed the calculation of SeHBV values, which were consistently positive and greater than 1 for both the $PaHgSe_2$ group (*P. amazonica*, a non-predatory species with higher C_{HgT}) and the $RvHgSe_2$ group (*R. vulpinus*, a predatory species with higher C_{HgT}). These results suggest that the mercury concentrations found in the muscle tissue of both *P. amazonica* and *R. vulpinus* pose a low health risk [12, 30–32]. Therefore, the findings presented here offer new insights into the attenuating effect of selenium on mercury's ability to generate oxidative species and potentially trigger oxidative stress.

4. Conclusions

The data reported in this study showed that the Hg:Se and Se:Hg molar ratios consistently reflected positive SeHBV values across both high and low mercury concentration groups in muscle tissue of both fish species studied. This strongly suggests that the organisms of both *P. amazonica* and *R. vulpinus* possess sufficient selenium reserves in their muscle tissue to mitigate the toxic effects of mercurial species. Furthermore, protein abundance analysis of the muscle proteome identified a limited number of proteins and/or enzymes with either *upregulation* or *downregulation*. Notably, the group with higher C_{HgT} (which also exhibited higher C_{SeT}) compared with the group with lower $C_{Hg}T$, displayed a reduced number of unique proteins. It can thus be inferred that selenium could be mitigating the negative impact of mercury on the function of these proteins and/or enzymes by forming [Se:Hg] inert complexes with the structures of these macromolecules. The observed correlations between SOD, CAT, and GPx enzyme activities, and LPO concentrations were stronger with C_{SeT} than with C_{HgT}. This finding suggests that oxidative stress caused by mercurial species does not occur in the muscle tissue of *P. amazonica* and *R. vulpinus*. Collectively, these insights indicate that the consumption of *P. amazonica* and *R. vulpinus* muscle tissue as a protein source by traditional Amazonian populations, apparently, does not present a risk of mercury contamination. To further strengthen these findings, future metalloproteomic studies are recommended. Specifically, identifying Hg and Se species in Hg/Se-associated protein spots in the muscle proteome of these fish, using a combination of two-dimensional electrophoresis (2D PAGE) with GFAAS-LC-MS/MS, would provide greater robustness to the data reported in this study.

Acknowledgements

Funding: This research was supported by São Paulo Research Foundation—FAPESP, Processes: 2021/01527-9 (Izabela da Cunha Bataglioli), 2022/04961-4 (Beatriz Miotto); 2021/09344-0 and 2023/01023-6 (Victor Diego Faria); 2017/09466-3 and 2019/02538-4 (Pedro de Magalhães Padilha); National Council for Scientific and Technological Development—CNPq, Processes: 306440/2022-9, 408179/2022-8 and 404404/2023-5 (Pedro de Magalhães Padilha); CAPES-Print AUXPE-Process: 88881.3107432018-0.1 (Pedro de Magalhães Padilha); Financier of Studies and Projects—FINEP, Process: 0282/19 (Pedro de Magalhães Padilha).

Conflicts of interest

The authors declare that they have no known competing financial interests or personal.

Data availability statement

The datasets generated and analyzed during the current study are available in the UNESP Institutional Repository. https://repositorio.unesp.br/home.

Declaration of ethics approval

The protocols used in this research were approved by Chico Mendes Institute for Biodiversity Conservation and Authorization and Information System on Biodiversity

(ICMBio; Ref. SISBIO 43890-1) and the Committee on Ethics in the Use of Animals (CEUA), protocol number no. 0316/2023.

Supplementary information

Additional supplementary information may be found in the supplementary information tab for this chapter: https://drive.google.com/file/d/1MfRdnz3031WXPsP0vkWWaUNXfvNNcrpf/view?usp=sharing

Author details

Izabela da Cunha Bataglioli[1], José Cavalcante Souza Vieira[2], Victor Diego Faria[2], Ronaldo de Almeida[3], Joyce Andrade da Silva[1], Luane B. Gonçalves Andrade[1], Felipe Dalmazzo Cirinêu[2], Luiz Fabrício Zara[4], Marília Afonso Rabelo Buzalaf[5], Jiri Adamec[6] and Pedro de Magalhães Padilha[1,2]*

1 School of Veterinary Medicine and Animal Science, São Paulo State University (UNESP), Botucatu, São Paulo, Brazil

2 Institute of Biosciences, São Paulo State University (UNESP), Botucatu, São Paulo, Brazil

3 Federal University of Rondonia, Wolfgang C. Pfeiffer Environmental Biogeochemistry Laboratory, Porto Velho, RO, Brazil

4 University of Brasília (UNB), College of Planaltina, Distrito Federal, Brazil

5 Bauru Dentistry College, University of São Paulo, (USP), Bauru, Brazil

6 School of Medicine, Louisiana State University Health Sciences Center (LSUHSC), Louisiana, New Orleans, USA

*Address all correspondence to: pedro.padilha@unesp.br

References

[1] Scheuhammer A, Braune B, Chan HM, Frouin H, Krey A, Letcher R, et al. Recent progress on our understanding of the biological effects of mercury in fish and wildlife in the Canadian Arctic. Science of the Total Environment. 2015;**509**:91-103

[2] Bosch AC, O'Neill B, Sigge GO, Kerwath SE, Hoffman LC. Mercury accumulation in yellowfin tuna (Thunnus albacares) with regards to muscle type, muscle position and fish size. Food Chemistry. 2016;**190**:351-356

[3] Yang L, Zhang Y, Wang F, Luo Z, Guo S, Strahle U. Toxicity of mercury: Molecular evidence. Chemosphere. 2020;**245**:125586

[4] Bank MS, Frantzen S, Duinker A, Amouroux D, Tessier E, Nedreaas K, et al. Rapid temporal decline of mercury in Greenland halibut (Reinhardtius hippoglossoides). Environmental Pollution. 2021;**289**:117843

[5] Wiech M, Bienfait AM, Silva M, Barre J, Sele V, Bank MS, et al. Organ-specific mercury stable isotopes, speciation and particle measurements reveal methylmercury detoxification processes in Atlantic Bluefin tuna. Journal of Hazardous Materials. 2024;**473**:134699

[6] Silva SF, Lima ML. Mercury in fish marketed in the Amazon triple frontier and health risk assessment. Chemosphere. 2020;**248**:125989

[7] Silva SF, Oliveira DC, Pereira JPG, Simone Pinto Castro SP, Costa BNS, Lima ML. Seasonal variation of mercury in commercial fishes of the Amazon triple frontier, Western Amazon Basin. Ecological Indicators. 2019;**106**:105549

[8] Ralston NVC, Raymond LJ. Mercury's neurotoxicity is characterized by its disruption of selenium biochemistry. Biochimica et Biophysica Acta (BBA) - General Subjects. 2018;**1862**:2405-2416

[9] Tomza-Marciniak A, Pilarczyk B, Drozd R, Pilarczyk R, Juszczak-Czasnoj CM, Havryliak V, et al. Selenium and mercury concentrations, Se:Hg molar ratios and their effect on the antioxidant system in wild mammals. Journal of Trace Elements in Medicine and Biology. 2023;**322**:121234

[10] Mellingen RM, Myrmel LS, Rasinger JD, Lie KK, Bernhard A, Madsen L, et al. Selenomethionine reduce mercury tissue levels and modulate methylmercury induced proteomic and transcriptomic alterations in hippocampi of adolescent BALB/c mice. International Journal Molecular Science. 2022;**23**:12242

[11] Gochfeld M, Joanna Burger J. Mercury interactions with selenium and sulfur and the relevance of the Se:Hg molar ratio to fish consumption advic. Environmental Science and Pollution Research. 2021;**28**:18407-18420

[12] Lino AS, Kasper D, Guida YS, Thomaz JR, Malm O. Mercury and selenium in fishes from the Tapajos River in the Brazilian Amazon: An evaluation of human exposure. Journal of Trace Elements in Medicine and Biology. 2018;**48**:196-201

[13] Mounicou S, Szpunar J, Lobinski R. Metallomics: The concept and methodology. Chemical Society Reviews. 2009;**38**:1119-1138

[14] Szpunar J. Advances in analytical methodology for bioinorganic speciation analysis: Metallomics, metalloproteomics

and heteroatom-tagged proteomics and metabolomics. Analyst. 2005;**130**(4): 442-465

[15] Garcia JS, Magalhães CS, Arruda MAZ. Trends in metal-binding and metalloproteins analysis. Talanta. 2006;**69**:1-15

[16] Bittarello AC, Vieira JCS, Braga CP, de Paula Araújo WL, da Cunha Bataglioli I, da Silva JM, et al. Characterization of molecular biomarkers of mercury exposure to muscle tissue of Plagioscion squamosissimus and Colossoma macropomum from the Amazon region. Food Chemistry. 2019;**276**:247-254

[17] Pacheco AC, Bartolette R, Caluca JF, De Castro ALM, Albrecht MP, Caramaschi EP. Dinâmica alimentar de Rhaphiodon vulpinus Agassiz, 1829 (Teleostei, Cynodontidae) no alto Rio Tocantins (GO) em relação ao represamento pela UHE Serra da Mesa. Biota Neotropica. 2009;**9**(3):77-84

[18] Malabarba L, Malabarba MC. Phylogeny and classification of Neotropical fish. In: Baldisserotto B, Cyrino J, Urbinati E, editors. Biology and Physiology of Freshwater Neotropical Fish. 1st ed. Jaboticabal: FUNEP; 2014. pp. 1-12

[19] Silva FA, Neves RCF, Quintero-Pinto LG, Padilha CCF, JorgeSMA,BarrosMM,et al.Determination of selenium by GFAAS in slurries of fish feces to estimate the bioavailability of this micronutrient in feed used in pisciculture. Chemosphere. 2007;**68**:1542-1547

[20] Moraes PM, Santos FA, Cavecci B, Padilha CCF, Vieira JVS, Roldam PS, et al. GFAAS determination of mercury in muscle samples of fish from Amazon, Brazil. Food Chemistry. 2013;**141**:2614-2617

[21] Bittencourt LO, Chemelo VS, Aragão WAB, Puty B, Dionizio A, Teixeira FB, et al. From molecules to behavior in long-term inorganic mercury intoxication: Unraveling proteomic features in cerebellar neurodegeneration of rats. International Journal of Molecular Sciences. 2021;**23**:111

[22] Wang T, Cai X, Li J, Xie L. Proteomics analysis in myocardium of spontaneously hypertensive rats. Scientific Reports. 2023;**13**:276

[23] Erden M, Bor NM. Changes of reduced glutathion, glutathion reductase, and glutathione peroxidase afterradiation in Guinea pigs. Biochemical Medecine. 1984;**31**:217-227

[24] Beutler E. Red Cell Metabolism: A Manual of Biochemical a Methods. New York: Grune&Stron; 1975

[25] Crouch RK, Gandy SE, Kimsey G, Galbraith RA, Galbraith GMP, Buse MG. The inhibition of islet superoxide dismutase by diabetogenic drugs. Diabetes. 1981;**30**:235-241

[26] Jiang ZY, Woollard ACS, Wolff SP. Lipid hydroperoxides measurement by oxidation of Fe^{2+} in the presence of xylenol orange comparison with the TBA assay and an iodometric method. Lipids. 1991;**26**:853-856

[27] Souza LRR, Zannata MBT, da Silva IA, Silva da Veiga MAM. Mercury determination in soil and sludge samples by HR CS GFAAS: Comparison of sample preparation procedures and chemical modifiers. Journal of Analytical Atomic Spectrometry. 2018;**33**:1477-1485

[28] Gomez-Nieto B, Gismera MJ, Sevilla MT, Procopio JR. Direct solid sampling of biological species for the rapid determination of selenium by high-resolution continuum source

graphite furnace atomic absorption spectrometry. Analytica Chimica Acta. 2022;**1202**:339637

[29] Anna Bizo'n A, Chojdak-Łukasiewicz J, Budrewicz S, Pokryszko-Dragan A, Piwowar A. Exploring the relationship between antioxidant enzymes, oxidative stress markers, and clinical profile in relapsing–remitting multiple sclerosis. Antioxidants. 2023;**12**:1638

[30] Kaneko J, Ralston N, N. Selenium and mercury in pelagic fish in the central North Pacific near Hawaii. Biological Trace Element Research. 2007;**119**(2007):242-254

[31] Ralston NVC, Ralston CR, Raymond LJ. Selenium health benefit values: Updated criteria for mercury risk assessments. Biological Trace Element Research. 2016;**171**:262-269

[32] Ralston NVC, Kaneko JJ, Raymond LJ. Selenium health benefit values provide a reliable index of seafood benefits vs. risks. Journal of Trace Elements in Medicine and Biology. 2019;**55**:50-57

[33] Pearson RG. Hard and soft acids and bases. Journal of the American Chemical Society. 1963;**85**:3533-3539

[34] UniProt, 2024. Universal Protein Resource (UniProt) [WWW Document]. 2024. Available from: http://www.uniprot.org/ [Accessed: November 03, 2024]

[35] Bittarello AC, Vieira JCS, Braga CP, Bataglioli IC, Oliveira G, Rocha LC, et al. Metalloproteomic approach of mercury-binding proteins in liver and kidney tissues of *Plagioscion squamosissimus* (corvina) and *Colossoma macropomum* (tambaqui) from Amazon region: Possible identification of mercury contamination biomarkers. Science of the Total Environment. 2020;**711**:134547

[36] Vieira JCS, Braga CP, Oliveira G, Padilha CCF, Moraes PM, Zara LF, et al. Mercury exposure: Protein biomarkers of mercury exposure in Jaraqui fish from the Amazon region. Biological Trace Element Research. 2018;**183**:164-171

[37] Bataglioli IC, Vieira JCS, Queiroz JV, Fernandes MS, Bittarello AC, Braga CP, et al. Physiological and functional aspects of metal-binding protein associated with mercury in the liver tissue of pirarucu (Arapaima gigas) from the Brazilian Amazon. Chemosphere. 2019;**236**:124320

[38] Hussmann M, Schulte D, Weischer S, Carlantoni C, Nakajima H, Mochizuki N, et al. Svep1 is a binding ligand of Tie1 and affects specific aspects of facial lymphatic development in a Vegfc-independent manner. eLife. 2023;**12**:e82969

[39] Almeida EC, Faria VD, Cirinêu FD, Santiago MGA, Miotto B, Vieira JCS, et al. Metalloproteomic investigation of Hg-binding proteins in renal tissue of rats exposed to mercury chloride. International Journal Molecular Science. 2024;**25**(1):164

[40] Vieira JCS, Braga CP, de Queiroz JV, Cavecci-Mendonça B, de Oliveira G, de Freitas NG, et al. The effects of mercury exposure on Amazonian fishes: An investigation of potential biomarkers. Chemosphere. 2023;**316**(137779):3

[41] Bataglioli ICB, Queiroz JV, Vieira JCS, Cavalline NG, Braga PB, Buzalaf MAR, et al. Mercury metalloproteomic profile in muscle tissue of Arapaima gigas from the Brazilian Amazon. Environmental Monitoring and Assessment. 2022;**194**:705-716

[42] Hake SB, David Allis C. Histone H3 variants and their potential role in indexing mammalian genomes: The "H3 barcode hypotheses". Proceedings of the National Academy of Science. 2006;**103**:6428-6435

[43] Santiago MGA, Faria VD, Cirinêu FD, da Silva LLLQ, Almeida EC, Cavallini GC, et al. Metalloproteomic approach to liver tissue of rats exposed to mercury. Chemosphere. 2023;**312**:137222

[44] Queiroz JV, Vieira JCS, Oliveira G, Braga CP, Bataglioli IC, Silva JM, et al. Identification of biomarkers of mercury contamination in brachyplatystoma filamentosum of the Madeira River, Brazil, using metalloproteomic strategies. Biological Trace Element Research. 2019;**187**:291-300

[45] Cavecci-Mendonça B, Vieira JCS, Lima PM, Lima AL, Buzalaf MAR, Zara LF, et al. Study of proteins with mercury in fish from the Amazon region. Food Chemistry. 2020;**309**:125460

Chapter 6

Perspective Chapter: Comprehensive Overview of Electrochemical Sensors – Advanced Functional Materials, Surface Modification Techniques, Emerging Applications, and Computational Modeling

Jassem Wannassi, Gassoumi Bouzid, Mohamed Achraf Bouicha, Nicole Jaffrezic-Renault, Eduardo Alberto Lopez Maldonado and Houcine Barhoumi

Abstract

Recent advances in electrochemical sensors have considerably enhanced their performance and broadened their application scope. The introduction of advanced functional materials such as nanostructures, metal-organic frameworks (MOFs), and graphene-based composites has improved sensor sensitivity, selectivity, and stability, enabling the detection of trace-level analytes. Innovative surface modification strategies, such as electrode functionalization, bioconjugation, and self-assembled monolayers (SAMs), have optimized sensor interfaces, improving performance and biorecognition capabilities. These advancements have led to the emergence of new applications in point-of-care diagnostics, smart wearable biosensors, food safety monitoring, and environmental remediation. The continuous integration of novel materials and fabrication techniques is driving the evolution of electrochemical sensors toward more sensitive, selective, and cost-effective devices for a wide range of practical and societal challenges. The density functional theory (DFT), incorporating the quantum theory of atom in molecules (QTAIM) and non-covalent interaction (NCI) analysis, has been employed to investigate ZIF-8 as a model system. These approaches underscore the efficacy of these theoretical methods in complementing experimental findings for sensor device applications.

Keywords: chemical sensors, electrochemical performance, functional materials, surface modification, DFT

1. Introduction

Electrochemical sensors have become essential analytical tools for detecting various chemical and biological substances, thanks to their high sensitivity, rapid response, and cost-effectiveness [1, 2]. These sensors convert chemical interactions at the electrode surface into measurable electrical signals, enabling both qualitative and quantitative analysis of target analytes [3]. Operating on electrochemical transduction mechanisms such as amperometry, voltammetry, potentiometry, and electrochemical impedance spectroscopy (EIS), each technique offers distinct advantages based on the application [4]. The demand for electrochemical sensors has surged in environmental monitoring, biomedical diagnostics, and food safety, where they provide portable, real-time detection of contaminants, biomarkers, and pollutants [5]. Their ability to detect trace-level substances makes them an attractive alternative to conventional methods like atomic absorption spectroscopy (AAS) and inductively coupled plasma mass spectrometry (ICP-MS) [6].

Recent innovations in materials, such as nanomaterials, conductive polymers, and metal-organic frameworks (MOFs), have significantly enhanced sensor performance, particularly in terms of sensitivity, selectivity, and stability. Additionally, electrode surface modification and functionalization strategies have further improved their efficiency [7–11]. Integration with digital technologies, like artificial intelligence and wireless communication, is expanding the applications of electrochemical sensors in real-time monitoring and data analysis [12–15]. Despite these advancements, challenges like electrode fouling, stability, and interference remain, requiring continued research in material engineering and electrode optimization [16–18]. The latest developments in electrochemical sensors explore material innovations, surface modification strategies, and their broadening applications, particularly in detecting heavy metals and biomolecules, aiming to address global challenges in environmental pollution, public health, and food safety [19, 20]. To validate the detection processes of heavy metals, gases, and organic dyes, the density functional theory (DFT) emerges as a highly effective method for elucidating selective binding sites, investigating the forces that underpin a compound's stability, and confirming the sensing capabilities of each compound for target entities. The DFT approach, which encompasses the quantum theory of molecules (QTAIM) and non-covalent interactions (NCI), provides a sophisticated framework for interpreting experimental results and deepening our understanding of the sensor mechanism through straightforward schematic representations, offering a more comprehensive insight into sensing phenomena. We conclude with a DFT model for ZIF-8.

2. Electrochemical sensors: Principles and mechanisms

Electrochemical sensors function by converting a chemical reaction or binding event into an electrical signal, which is then analyzed to determine the concentration of the target analyte. These sensors are broadly classified into

- Amperometric sensors: Measure current as a function of analyte concentration.
- Potentiometric sensors: Measure potential changes at the working electrode.
- Impedimetric sensors: Measure changes in charge transfer resistance and capacitance at the electrode surface.

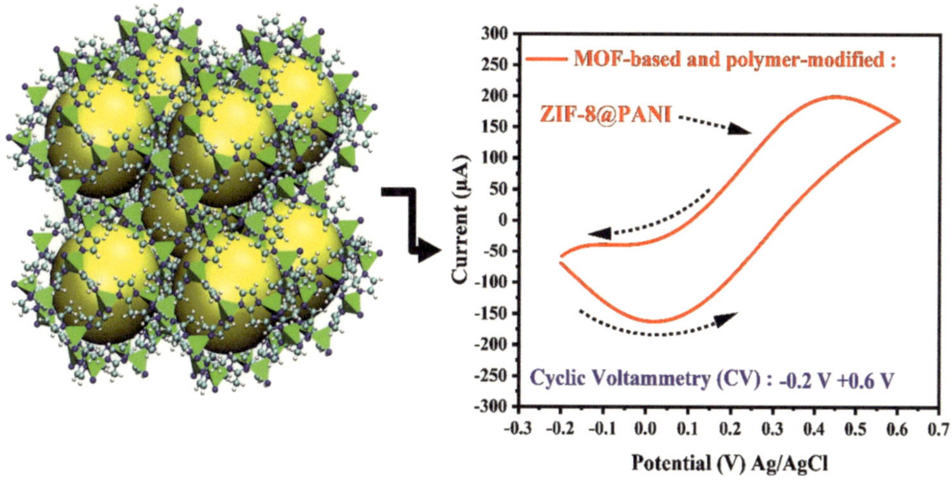

Figure 1.
MOF-based and polymer-modified electrodes.

The working principle of electrochemical sensors involves three key components

- Electrode material: Determines charge transfer efficiency and sensor stability.
- Recognition element: Enhances selectivity by selectively binding to the target analyte.

Transduction mechanism: Converts chemical interactions into an electrical signal, analyzed *via* techniques such as cyclic voltammetry (CV), differential pulse voltammetry (DPV), and electrochemical impedance spectroscopy (EIS).

MOF-based and polymer-modified electrodes demonstrate superior electrochemical performance due to their high surface area, controlled porosity, and functionalized active sites (**Figure 1**), which enhance analyte adsorption and charge transfer [21].

3. Functional materials in electrochemical sensors

The performance of electrochemical sensors is largely influenced by the choice of functional materials used in their construction. Recent research has focused on developing advanced materials that offer superior electrocatalytic properties, high surface area, and enhanced stability. Notable examples include: Nanostructured materials: The use of nanomaterials, such as carbon nanotubes (CNTs), graphene, and metal nanoparticles, has revolutionized electrochemical sensors. These materials exhibit excellent conductivity, a large surface area, and the ability to adsorb a variety of analytes, significantly improving sensor performance, particularly in voltammetric and amperometric applications. Metal-Organic Frameworks (MOFs): MOFs have gained significant attention due to their high porosity, tunable structures, and large surface areas, which provide enhanced interaction with target analytes. Materials like HKUST-1 and ZIF-8 have been widely explored for heavy metal ion detection, biosensing, and gas sensing applications. Their unique properties make them ideal for the construction of high-performance electrochemical sensors (**Figure 2**).

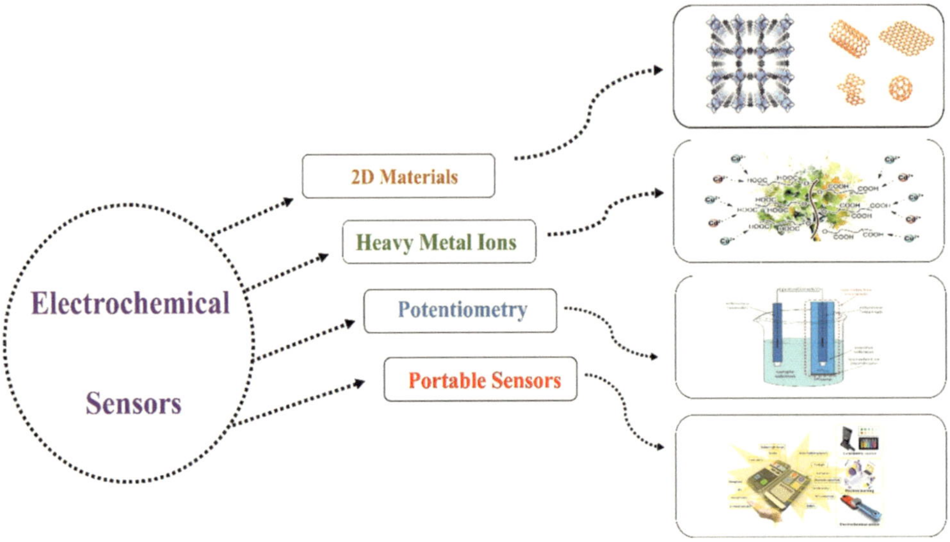

Figure 2.
Functional materials used in electrochemical sensors for enhanced performance and sensitivity.

Conducting polymers: Polymers such as polyaniline (PANI) and polypyrrole (PPy) are used to modify electrode surfaces, improving both the electrochemical properties and mechanical stability of sensors. The ability to tailor their electrical conductivity and surface reactivity makes them suitable for various sensing applications, including pH sensing, bio-detection, and toxin sensing. Hybrid Materials: The combination of different materials, such as MOFs with conducting polymers or graphene, has led to the creation of hybrid materials with enhanced properties. These composite materials often exhibit synergistic effects, such as improved electrical conductivity, chemical stability, and selectivity, which are essential for sensitive and reliable electrochemical sensing.

4. Surface modification strategies

Surface modification is essential for improving the performance of electrochemical sensors. By tailoring the electrode surface, researchers can enhance the interaction between the electrode and the analyte, improving both sensitivity and selectivity. Key surface modification strategies include: Electrode functionalization: This involves modifying the surface of electrodes with various functional groups to enhance analyte binding and detection. Self-assembled monolayers (SAMs) are commonly used to immobilize biorecognition elements such as enzymes, antibodies, or aptamers, allowing the sensor to selectively interact with target molecules. Nanostructuring of electrodes: Creating nanoscale features on electrode surfaces significantly increases the surface area and facilitates better electrode-analyte interactions. Techniques such as nanoparticle deposition and nanopatterning have led to sensors with superior sensitivity, particularly in biosensing and chemical detection. Bioconjugation and molecular imprinting: Bioconjugation involves the attachment of biomolecules to the electrode surface to create specific recognition sites, whereas molecular imprinting involves the creation of molecular cavities in the polymer matrix tailored for

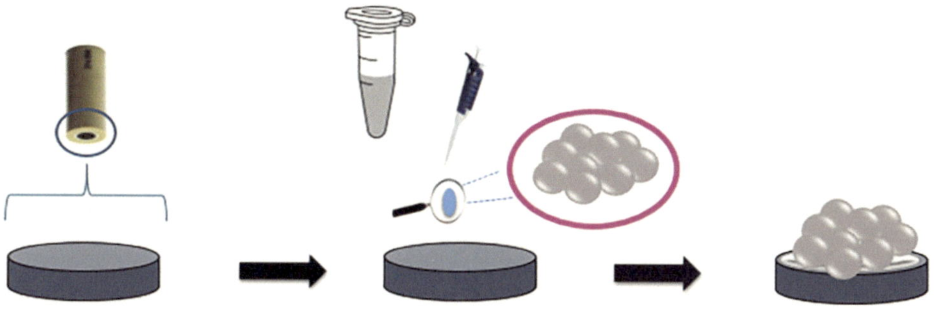

Figure 3.
Surface modification strategies for enhanced sensor performance.

specific analytes. Both strategies significantly enhance the selectivity and sensitivity of electrochemical sensors, making them particularly useful for toxin detection, biomarker sensing, and food safety applications. Layer-by-layer (LbL) assembly: The LbL technique allows for the precise control over the construction of multi-layered sensor surfaces, which can improve electrochemical response and selectivity. It is particularly useful for creating complex biosensors and chemical sensors (**Figure 3**).

Surface modification is essential for enhancing the sensitivity, selectivity, and stability of electrochemical sensors. Strategies such as electrode functionalization, nanostructuring, bioconjugation, and molecular imprinting improve analyte interaction and signal transduction. Materials like metal nanoparticles, carbon nanostructures, conducting polymers, and MOFs are commonly employed to optimize surface properties and electron transfer. Additionally, conducting polymers like polyaniline (PANI) and polypyrrole (PPy) provide excellent biocompatibility and signal amplification properties. Chemical grafting and self-assembled monolayers (SAMs) are also employed to introduce specific functional groups that enhance target analyte recognition. Furthermore, molecular imprinting techniques enable the creation of highly selective sensing surfaces for detecting specific molecules in complex samples. These surface modification strategies have led to significant advancements in electrochemical sensor technology, enabling the detection of ultra-low concentrations of environmental pollutants, biomolecules, and industrial contaminants with high precision and reliability.

5. Toxicology and relevance to electrochemical sensing

Toxicology is the scientific discipline that investigates the adverse effects of chemical substances on living organisms and the environment. It plays a crucial role in understanding the impact of contaminants such as heavy metals, pesticides, and organic pollutants, which pose significant risks even at trace levels. Electrochemical sensors have emerged as powerful tools in toxicological analysis, offering rapid, sensitive, and cost-effective detection of toxic agents in various matrices including water, food, and biological fluids. The integration of toxicological knowledge into sensor design enhances the development of devices tailored for early detection and quantification of hazardous substances, thus aiding in the prevention of exposure-related health effects.

Heavy metals such as lead (Pb^{2+}), cadmium (Cd^{2+}), and mercury (Hg^{2+}) are among the most concerning environmental toxins due to their high toxicity, persistence, and bioaccumulation in the food chain. Chronic exposure to these metals can lead to neurological, renal, and developmental disorders. Electrochemical sensors, especially those based on modified electrodes with nanostructured materials or MOFs, have shown great promise in detecting these toxicants at ultra-trace concentrations. Their high sensitivity and selectivity stem from the engineered surface functionalities that mimic biological interactions, making them particularly suitable for toxicological screening in environmental and clinical settings.

From a regulatory perspective, toxicological limits established by organizations such as the WHO, EPA, and EU are essential benchmarks in sensor development. Electrochemical sensors must be validated to reliably detect toxic substances below these permissible exposure limits. Moreover, real-sample testing in complex matrices (e.g., tap water, river water, and serum) is essential to demonstrate sensor applicability and robustness. By aligning with toxicological frameworks and thresholds, electrochemical sensors contribute not only to academic research but also to public health surveillance and environmental policy enforcement.

Figure 4 presents the differential pulse voltammetry (DPV) response for the simultaneous detection of Cd^{2+}, Pb^{2+}, Cu^{2+}, and Hg^{2+} ions using a ZIF-8@PANI-modified glassy carbon electrode (GCE) in 0.1 M acetate buffer solution. The voltammogram exhibits four distinct and well-separated peaks located approximately at −0.78, −0.50, −0.05, and + 0.20 V, corresponding to the reduction of Cd^{2+}, Pb^{2+}, Cu^{2+}, and Hg^{2+}, respectively. Among them, the Pb^{2+} peak shows the highest current intensity (~55 μA), indicating a strong interaction and high sensitivity of the modified electrode toward lead ions. The well-defined separation between peaks confirms the sensor's excellent selectivity and ability to detect multiple heavy metal ions simultaneously without signal overlap. The synergistic combination of ZIF-8, offering high surface area and porosity, with the conductive polymer PANI significantly enhances the electron transfer kinetics and adsorption

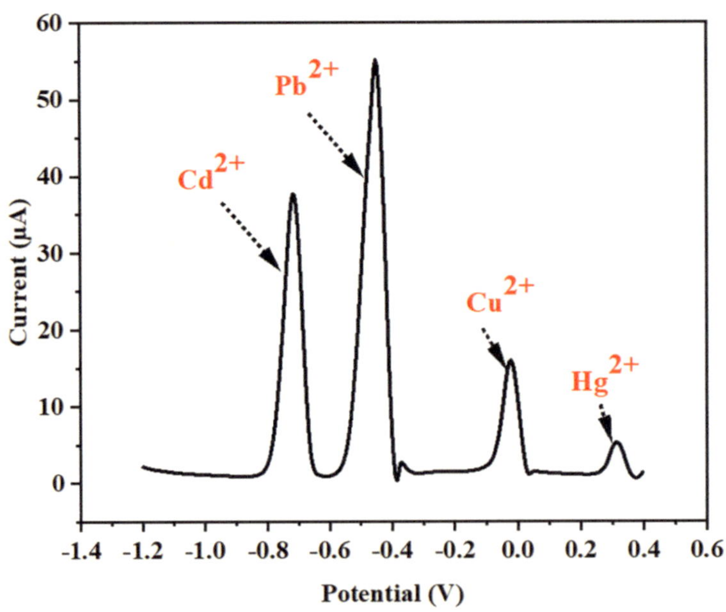

Figure 4.
Differential pulse voltammetry for simultaneous detection of Cd^{2+}, Pb^{2+}, Cu^{2+} and Hg^{2+} on ZIF-8@PANI/GCE in 0.1 M acetate buffer solution.

capacity, thereby improving the electrochemical performance of the sensor. From a toxicological perspective, the detection of these metal ions is critically important due to their severe effects on human health and the environment. Lead (Pb^{2+}) and mercury (Hg^{2+}) are known neurotoxins even at low concentrations, while cadmium (Cd^{2+}) is associated with kidney damage and carcinogenic risks. Copper (Cu^{2+}), though essential in trace amounts, becomes toxic in excess. The reliable and simultaneous detection of these ions is therefore essential for environmental monitoring and public health. Electrochemical sensing offers a highly attractive platform for this purpose due to its inherent advantages such as simplicity, low cost, portability, rapid response, and high sensitivity. The performance demonstrated in this figure highlights the potential of the ZIF-8@PANI/GCE sensor as an effective tool for real-time monitoring of toxic heavy metals in environmental samples.

6. Emerging applications

As electrochemical sensors continue to evolve, their applications are expanding into new and emerging areas. Some of the key applications include:

- Environmental Monitoring: Electrochemical sensors are increasingly used for monitoring air quality, water pollution, and heavy metal contamination. Techniques such as voltammetry and amperometry allow for the real-time detection of pollutants, heavy metals, and toxic substances in the environment. The ability to detect trace amounts of pollutants in real-time makes electrochemical sensors a powerful tool for environmental protection and sustainability.

- Biomedical Diagnostics: Electrochemical sensors are widely used in point-of-care diagnostics, where they offer rapid, cost-effective, and non-invasive detection of biomarkers, glucose, and other metabolites. Electrochemical biosensors have proven to be essential tools for early disease detection, such as for cancer biomarkers, infection monitoring, and diabetes management.

- Food Safety and Quality Control: Electrochemical sensors offer a promising solution for detecting contaminants and pathogens in food products. Their portability, sensitivity, and ability to detect multiple analytes in real-time make them ideal for use in food safety applications, where rapid analysis is critical.

- Wearable and Smart Sensors: The integration of flexible electrochemical sensors into wearable devices has opened new avenues for continuous health monitoring, particularly in the context of chronic disease management and personalized medicine. These sensors enable real-time tracking of glucose levels, hydration, and other physiological parameters, offering a more convenient and affordable approach to healthcare.

- Industrial Process Control: Electrochemical sensors are being utilized for industrial monitoring in sectors such as chemical production, energy storage, and pharmaceutical manufacturing. These sensors allow for precise and real-time monitoring of chemical processes, enabling better quality control and process optimization.

Electrochemical sensors are gaining increasing attention in advanced detection technologies due to their high sensitivity, rapid response, and cost-effectiveness. These

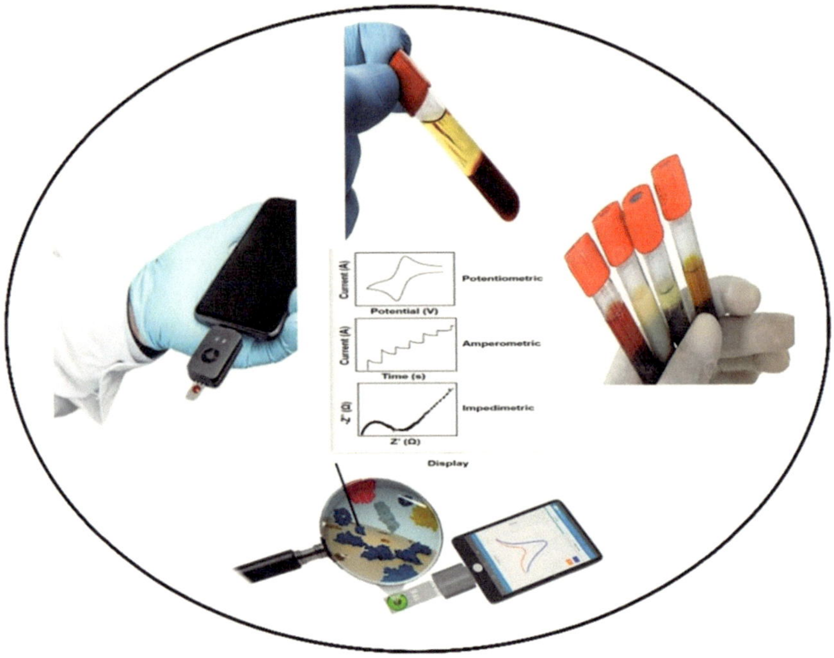

Figure 5.
Emerging applications of electrochemical sensors in advanced detection technologies.

sensors have evolved beyond traditional applications and are now being integrated into diverse fields such as environmental monitoring, biomedical diagnostics, food safety, and industrial quality control (as indicated in **Figure 5**). Recent advancements in nanomaterials, metal-organic frameworks (MOFs), and functionalized electrodes have significantly enhanced their selectivity and detection limits. In medical diagnostics, electrochemical sensors enable real-time monitoring of biomarkers for early disease detection, while in environmental analysis, they facilitate the accurate quantification of heavy metals and organic pollutants in water and soil. Moreover, the integration of electrochemical sensors with portable and wireless technologies has opened new possibilities for on-site and point-of-care testing, offering practical solutions for real-world challenges. As research progresses, the continued development of miniaturized, multi-analyte, and self-powered electrochemical sensors is expected to revolutionize analytical detection technologies, making them more accessible and efficient.

6.1 Regulatory considerations and clinical translation

Despite significant progress in wearable and biomedical electrochemical sensors, transitioning from laboratory prototypes to clinical or commercial devices requires navigating rigorous regulatory pathways [3]. For instance, approval by regulatory bodies such as the U.S. Food and Drug Administration (FDA) or European Conformity (CE) marking involves comprehensive validation of safety, biocompatibility, analytical performance, and long-term stability. In addition to clinical trials, adherence to Good Manufacturing Practices (GMP) and ISO standards for medical devices is essential. These requirements pose challenges related to reproducibility, sensor miniaturization, and patient-specific variability. Nonetheless, addressing these regulatory and translational hurdles is critical for advancing electrochemical biosensors into widespread clinical use and establishing their reliability in real-world healthcare settings [3].

6.2 Case study: Portable electrochemical sensor for on-site heavy metal detection

A practical example of real-world deployment is the use of a portable electrochemical sensor based on a ZIF-8@PANI-modified glassy carbon electrode for the simultaneous detection of Pb^{2+}, Cd^{2+}, Cu^{2+}, and Hg^{2+} in river and tap water samples. The sensor was integrated into a handheld voltammetric analyzer and tested on-site near industrial discharge zones. Differential pulse voltammetry (DPV) measurements revealed well-resolved peaks for all target ions, with recovery rates ranging from 94–102% and relative standard deviations below 5%, confirming the sensor's reliability in complex matrices. This case illustrates how lab-developed sensors can be effectively translated into field-deployable systems for environmental monitoring, with the potential to support rapid decision-making and regulatory compliance.

7. Density functional theory (DFT) in electrochemical sensor design

Density Functional Theory (DFT) is a computational quantum mechanical method that describes the electronic structure of atoms, molecules, and materials by solving Schrödinger's equation in an approximate yet computationally efficient manner [22]. Unlike traditional wavefunction-based methods, DFT expresses the system's energy as a functional of electron density ($\rho(r)$), significantly reducing computational complexity.

7.1 Adsorption behavior and surface interaction studies

DFT is widely used to predict the binding energy and orientation of analytes on modified electrode surfaces. By analyzing adsorption configurations, researchers can:

- Identify favorable binding sites on MOFs, conducting polymers, and nanomaterials.
- Optimize functional groups that enhance selectivity.
- Investigate hydrogen bonding, π–π interactions and metal coordination effects.

7.2 Electronic structure and charge transfer mechanisms

Understanding charge distribution and electron transfer at the electrode-analyte interface is critical for designing high-performance sensors [23]. DFT-based density of states (DOS) and Bader charge analysis can:

- Determine how electrons transfer between the electrode and the analyte.
- Predict the rate of electrochemical reactions based on band alignment.
- Explain how dopants and composite materials influence conductivity.

7.3 Development of novel sensor materials

By screening materials computationally before synthesis, DFT accelerates the development of novel sensor materials [24]. This approach enables:

- Virtual screening of MOF candidates for enhanced adsorption and electron transfer.

- Predicting the effects of functionalization on sensor selectivity.

Identifying hybrid materials with synergistic properties.

7.4 Limitations and challenges in DFT modeling

While DFT offers powerful insight into the electronic structure and surface interactions of sensing materials, it also presents several limitations. The accuracy of DFT predictions heavily depends on the choice of exchange-correlation functional; commonly used generalized gradient approximation (GGA) functionals may fail to capture weak van der Waals interactions unless dispersion corrections (e.g., DFT-D3) are included. Additionally, most DFT simulations are performed under vacuum or idealized conditions, which may not accurately reflect the complexities of electrochemical environments such as solvent effects, pH variations, or electrode potentials. Furthermore, DFT is fundamentally a static method and cannot inherently capture dynamic processes like real-time charge transfer, ion diffusion, or electrochemical kinetics unless coupled with time-dependent DFT (TD-DFT) or molecular dynamics (MD) simulations. These limitations underscore the need to interpret DFT results alongside experimental data and to continue developing multiscale modeling approaches for more comprehensive sensor design.

8. Application of DFT on ZIF-8 as a model system

Herein, density functional theory (DFT) modeling and non-covalent interactions have been employed to enhance our experimental understanding of the sensor mechanism of ZIF-8 for selective detection of CO_2 and CH_4 gases [25, 26]. Utilizing the DFT-D3/B3LYP/LanL2DZ [27, 28] level of theory *via* the Gaussian09 package [29], we optimized each complex, with parameters fixed in the GaussView 6 interface [30]. The NCI index, visualized through color coding, elucidates the types and nature of all interactions responsible for the stability of gases at each binding site. This tool is generated using the VMD package [31]. **Figure 6** illustrates that the CO_2 is positioned at the center of the ZIF-cavity, equidistant from four symmetric carbon atoms at distances of 3.89, 281, 3.91, and 3.60 Å, respectively. Regarding the CH_4@MOF, it has been determined that the gas is effectively stabilized within the cavity center at distances from carbon atoms measuring 3.10, 2.81, 3.18, and 3.14 Å, respectively. Both gases appear to be nearly localized at the center of the ZIF-8 cavity, underscoring the efficacy of the computational method employed. The NCI analysis reveals that the CO_2 and CH_4 gases are well stabilized through van der Waals interactions (indicated by the green color). This finding demonstrates the potential of this compound for efficient gas detection applications. Moreover, this discovery paves the way for exploring this green material in other fields, such as biological applications and nano-electronic devices.

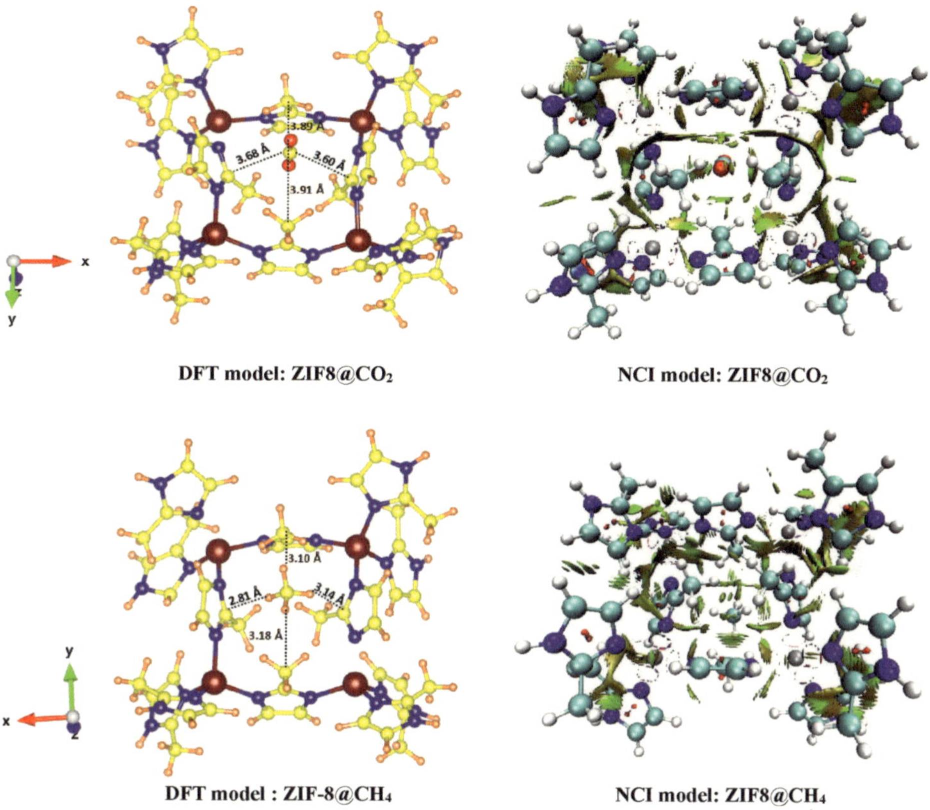

Figure 6.
Schematic representation of CO_2 and CH_4 gas sensing using DFT and NCI, featuring ZIF-8 as model.

9. Future perspectives in DFT-based sensor design

- AI-Driven DFT Simulations: Machine learning can accelerate material screening by predicting optimal electrode compositions for various analytes.
- Time-Dependent DFT (TD-DFT): Can be used to investigate dynamic charge transfer processes in real-time.
- Beyond Standard Functionals: Hybrid and GW approximations offer more accurate descriptions of electron correlation effects in sensor materials.
- Multiscale Modeling: Combining DFT with Molecular Dynamics (MD) can provide a more realistic representation of electrode-electrolyte interfaces.

10. Conclusion

Recent advancements in electrochemical sensors, particularly in the areas of functional materials and surface modification strategies, have paved the way for a new generation of highly sensitive, selective, and versatile sensors. These innovations have expanded the applicability of electrochemical sensors into emerging fields such as wearable health monitoring, food safety, and environmental protection, while also improving their performance in traditional applications such as biomedical diagnostics and chemical detection. As the field continues to evolve, the integration of novel materials and cutting-edge fabrication techniques will likely drive further progress in electrochemical sensor technology, opening new possibilities for real-time, on-site, and cost-effective detection across a range of industries. To enhance our understanding the sensor mechanism between two systems, the DFT and NCI methods has proven to be exceptionally well-suited for advanced experimental applications.

Acknowledgements

The authors express their gratitude to the PHC-UTIQUE project (grant number 24G1208), the Directorate General for Scientific Research (DGRS) and the Tunisian Ministry of Higher Education and Scientific Research (LR11ES55) for their partial support of this work.

Author details

Jassem Wannassi[1], Gassoumi Bouzid[1*], Mohamed Achraf Bouicha[2], Nicole Jaffrezic-Renault[3], Eduardo Alberto Lopez Maldonado[4*] and Houcine Barhoumi[1]

1 Laboratory of Interfaces and Advanced Materials, Faculty of Sciences, University of Monastir, Monastir, Tunisia

2 Laboratory of Physical Chemistry of Materials (LR01ES19), University of Monastir, Faculty of Sciences of Monastir, Avenue de l'environnement, Monastir, Tunisia

3 Institute of Analytical Sciences, University of Lyon, Villeurbanne, France

4 Faculty of Chemical Sciences and Engineering, Autonomous University of Baja California, Mexico

*Address all correspondence to: gassoumibouzid2016@gmail.com; elopez92@uabc.edu.mx

References

[1] Wannassi J et al. Electrochemical sensors based on metal-organic framework and conductive polymer HKUST-1@ PANI for high-performance detection of lead ions. Journal of the Electrochemical Society. 2023;**170**(11):117504

[2] Moumen Y et al. Green synthesis of ZIF-8 combined with ruthenium nanoparticles for enhanced electrochemical detection of dopamine. Journal of the Electrochemical Society. 2025;**172**(2):027511

[3] Wannassi J et al. A high-performance electrochemical sensor based on Ni-Pt bimetallic nanoparticles doped metal organic framework ZIF-8 for the detection of dopamine. ChemPlusChem. 2025;**90**(3):e202400734

[4] Wannassi J et al. Box-Behnken response surface design for the optimization of a high-performance electrochemical dopamine sensor based on novel nano-Ag doped Matériaux Institut Lavoisier metal-organic framework 101 (MIL-101-Cr) composite modified glassy carbon electrode. Journal of the Electrochemical Society. 2024;**171**(9):097511

[5] Essousi H et al. Electrochemical sensor of oxytetracycline based on molecularly imprinted poly (3, 4-ethylenedioxythiophene)/MXene on graphene screen printed electrode. Microchemical Journal. 2025;**215**:114425

[6] Hedau B, Ha T-J. Post-synthesis surface modification of Cu/Zr metal azolate framework: A pathway to highly sensitive electrochemical biosensors for atrazine detection. Analytica Chimica Acta. 2025;**1337**:343547

[7] Choudhury S et al. A surface modified laser-induced graphene based flexible biosensor for multiplexed sweat analysis. Journal of Materials Chemistry B. 2025;**13**(1):274-287

[8] Hao X et al. Recent advancements in electrochemical sensors based on MOFs and their derivatives. Small. 2025;**21**(4):2408624

[9] Fathi M. An update review on ionic liquids applications in electrochemical sensors. Journal of Chemical, Biological and Medicinial Sciences. 2025;**1**(4):167-173

[10] Devi WS et al. Non-enzymatic g-C3N4 supported CuO derived-biochar based electrochemical sensors for trace level detection of malathion. Biosensors and Bioelectronics. 2025;**267**:116808

[11] Lu Y et al. New cosolvent-dependent electrochemical sensing behavior of a pair of isostructural ionic nickel (II) coordination polymers. Journal of Molecular Structure. 2025;**1319**:139569

[12] Tian S et al. MnO2 nanoparticles enhance the activity of the Zr-MOF matrix electrochemical sensor for efficiently identifying ultra-trace tetracycline residues in food. Microchimica Acta. 2025;**192**(1):1-11

[13] Tian H et al. Electrochemical sensing fibers for wearable health monitoring devices. Biosensors and Bioelectronics. 2024;**246**:115890

[14] Li B et al. Recent advance of nanomaterials modified electrochemical sensors in the detection of heavy metal ions in food and water. Food Chemistry. 2024;**440**:138213

[15] Li Y et al. Recent advances in molecularly imprinted polymer-based electrochemical sensors. Biosensors and Bioelectronics. 2024;**249**:116018

[16] Jiang Y et al. Research progress on portable electrochemical sensors for detection of mycotoxins in food and environmental samples. Chemical Engineering Journal. 2024;**485**:149860

[17] Liu W et al. Electrochemical sensors for plant signaling molecules. Biosensors and Bioelectronics. 2024;**267**:116757

[18] Singh R et al. A review on recent trends and future developments in electrochemical sensing. ACS Omega. 2024;**9**(7):7336-7356

[19] Dourandish Z et al. Recent advances in electrochemical sensing of anticancer drug doxorubicin: A mini-review. Chemical Methodologies. 2024;**8**(4):293-315

[20] Nandi I, Rai SK, Chandra P. MOF-based nanocomposites as transduction matrices for optical and electrochemical sensing. Talanta. 2024;**266**:125124

[21] Ganesh P-S et al. Role of electron transfer between bare electrode and benzoguanamine to fabricate an electrochemical sensor for drugs: Theoretical and electrochemical approach. Microchemical Journal. 2024;**201**:110731

[22] Wannassi J et al. Highly selective and sensitive electrochemical sensor for mercury (II) detection using nickel (II)(bromophenyl) porphyrin on a glassy carbon electrode for environmental monitoring. Journal of the Electrochemical Society. 2025;**172**(4):047509

[23] Zhang X et al. Computational screening and experimental fabrication of MoSe2/3d–TMOS heterojunction for room-temperature gas sensor. Applied Surface Science. 2024;**654**:159465

[24] Achache M et al. Detection of paracetamol by a montmorillonite-modified carbon paste sensor: A study combining MC simulation, DFT computation and electrochemical investigations. Talanta. 2024;**274**:126027

[25] Belgacem CH, Missaoui N, Khalafalla MAH, Bouzid G, Kahri H, Bashal AH, et al. Synthesis of ultramicroporous zeolitic imidazolate framework ZIF-8 via solid state method using a minimum amount of deionized water for high greenhouse gas adsorption: A computational modeling. Journal of Environmental Chemical Engineering. 2024;**12**:112086. DOI: 10.1016/j.jece.2024.112086

[26] Missaoui N, Gassoumi B, Nasr S, Kaur H, Karayel A, Lopez-Maldonado EA, et al. Synergistic combination of experimental and theoretical studies on chlorinated volatile organic compound adsorption in highly microporous n-MOF-5 and amino-substituted n-MOF-5-NH2 nanocrystals synthesized via PEG soft-templating. Journal of Molecular Liquids. 2025;**418**:126716. DOI: 10.1016/j.molliq.2024.126716

[27] Liu D, He J, Wang R, Zhao Z, Dong Z, Bao Q, et al. Electron beam irradiation in collaboration with Bi-Fe MOFs for oxidation of bisphenol a and reduction of Cr(VI): Kinetics, DFT calculation and mechanism. Journal of Environmental Chemical Engineering. 2024;**12**:114945. DOI: 10.1016/j.jece.2024.114945

[28] de Almeida WL, Rodembusch FS, Ferreira NS, Caldas de Sousa V. Eco-friendly and cost-effective synthesis of ZnO nanopowders by tapioca-assisted sol-gel route. Ceramics International.

2020;**46**:10835-10842. DOI: 10.1016/j.ceramint.2020.01.095

[29] Frisch MJ, Trucks GW, Schlegel HB, Scuseria GE, Robb M, Cheeseman JR, et al. Gaussian 16, Revision A. 03. Wallingford CT 3: Gaussian, Inc.; 2016

[30] Roy DD, Todd AK, John MM. Gauss View 5.0.8. Wallingford: Gaussian Inc; 2009

[31] Humphrey W, Dalke A, Schulten K. VMD: Visual molecular dynamics. Journal of Molecular Graphics. 1996;**14**(33-38):27-28. DOI: 10.1016/0263-7855(96)00018-5